Dedication

To my wife Maureen, thank you for your love, support
and the warmth of your soul.

To my father for his inspiration and wisdom,
my mother (in memory of) for her divine guidance,
and my brothers and sisters for their encouragement.

Massage
Therapy
&
Medications

General Treatment Principles

RANDAL S. PERSAD Dip. Pharm., R.M.T.
FOREWORD BY DR. JOHN YATES Ph.D.

Massage Therapy & Medications
Randal S. Persad Dip. Pharm., R.M.T.
© Copyright 2001
2nd Printing 2002
3rd Printing 2004
4th Printing 2006
5th Printing 2007

To order copies, please contact:
Curties-Overzet Publications Inc.
330 Dupont Street, Suite 400
Toronto, Ontario
Canada M5R 1V9
Toll Free Phone: 1-888-649-5411
Fax: 416-923-8116
Website: www.sutherland-chan.com/copi
E-mail: copi@sutherland-chan.com

ISBN 978-0-9685256-2-3

The author and publisher have made every effort to ensure the accuracy of the contents of this book. However, appropriate sources should be consulted, especially for new or unfamiliar information. It is the responsibility of every practitioner to evaluate the appropriateness of a particular opinion in the context of actual clinical situations and with due consideration to new developments.

Acknowledgements

The writing of this book has spanned almost a decade; its beginnings are rooted back in the islands. To Lauren Lumkim, my teacher and mentor, thank you for believing in and encouraging me during those long hours of Pharmacy training.

There are many people who have encouraged and supported me in my writing. Thanks to the staff at Sutherland-Chan School & Teaching Clinic including Grace Chan, Eric Brown, Murray Pickering, Karen Friedl, Michael Bard, and Bruce McKinnon.

To the students and staff of the West Coast College of Massage Therapy, thank you for your questions, suggestions, and unsurpassed support during this writing adventure. Special thanks to John Ranney, Ron Garvock, Melba 'toast' Lewis, Natale Rao, Isabell MacDonald, Grace Dedinsky, Dr. Fernando Villsenior, Will Winram, Clifford Yip, Rich Ingram, Britta Hobkirk, Mike Dixon, and Steve Anderson. To Dr. Wayne Jakeman and associates, thank you for sharing and suggesting.

Many thanks to Paul Finch, Peter Becker, Geoff Harrison, and Jean Pascual for your help with text reading and proofing.

Finally, this project was made possible by the publisher and editor-in-chief Debra Curties, and the artistic creativity of Bev Ransom. I am especially grateful for your commitment, and appreciate the time you spent keeping me focused on deadlines and rewrites.

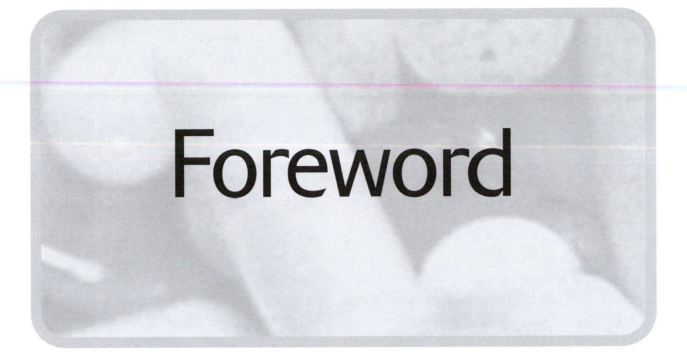

Foreword

The last two decades have witnessed several remarkable changes in the perceptions and practice of health care in North America. Dramatic new pharmaceutical agents have been developed, and they are being made available in a marketing environment where prescription medications to treat everything from high cholesterol to hypertension, anxiety, and impotence are being promoted directly to the public via television and magazine advertisements. Many powerful drugs are now also available over the counter or via the Internet without a prescription. At the same time, there has been an enormous groundswell of public interest in and utilization of alternative health care by all sectors of the population, including the postwar baby-boomers who have now reached middle age and are experiencing an increase in health problems of every sort. Many have come to regard non-conventional or alternative therapies as complementary to medical treatment, and are receiving such treatments while they are also under the care of a medical doctor for various medical conditions.

Massage is one of the most commonly used of the complementary therapies. It is well known for its value in relaxation and anxiety reduction, for treatment of many types of musculoskeletal pain and dysfunction, and for lessening discomforts associated with chronic disorders like arthritis and fibromyalgia. All of these conditions are also commonly treated by prescription or over-the-counter medications, and occur in people who may be using medications for other conditions at the same time. Massage therapists are more likely than ever before to regularly treat clients who are also using prescription and non-prescription medications.

Unfortunately, although most massage therapists are aware that their clients may be using medications, many lack formal training in their effects, their potential interactions with massage therapy modalities, and how to adapt massage treatments in these situations. Standards for training of massage therapists vary greatly throughout North America and rarely include a requirement for education about medications. As a result, few schools have addressed the need for training in basic pharmacology and the interactions between massage treatment and medications. This book fills a vital need by providing massage therapists with important basic information on the properties, mechanisms of action, and side effects of common medications, as well as how their presence in the client's body may influence treatment decisions and results.

One section has been devoted to the effects of medications on assessment results. Massage is performed for a broad spectrum of purposes that range from general relaxation and stress reduction, to treatment or rehabilitation of a number of injuries and conditions, to increased psychological comfort and enhanced sense of health and well-being. Massage therapists rely upon history taking, physical assessment, and palpation to determine which methods and techniques are most appropriate for the treatment of each client. The author has provided guidelines for good case history taking regarding medications, and discusses the various ways that concurrent drug use can affect assessment findings.

Randal Persad is ideally suited to have written this book. Originally trained as a pharmacist and employed by Lederle Laboratories, he subsequently became a massage therapist in 1991. While working in the hotel and spa industry, sports environment, and in chiropractic and rehabilitative settings, he noticed that many of his clientele were taking medications, and that the effects of their medications influenced their response to massage in ways that required him to adapt his treatments. Later, as an instructor at West Coast College of Massage Therapy in Vancouver, Canada, he was able to use this integrated knowledge of the actions of pharmaceuticals and the impacts of massage therapy to create guidelines for undergraduate students that encourage development of safe and effective treatment plans and minimize adverse reactions. Based on his unique background and teaching experience, he was asked to develop the medications component of the curriculum guideline for the College of Massage Therapists of British Columbia.

Mr. Persad has brought this rich background of knowledge and experience to bear on the task of providing a practical and useful introduction to pharmacological concepts, principles, and terminology. His discussion takes a complex subject and makes it easy to grasp and apply in clinical practice. He also provides the therapist with tools for better communication with doctors, pharmacists, and other health care professionals. Both general guidelines for working with clients who are taking medications and specific guidelines for working around injection sites and implants have been provided.

This book will help therapists develop the skills to interpret and understand the package information of common drugs and to recognize those drug effects that can potentially influence a massage treatment. That information can then be interpreted as it applies to manual therapy, and used to adapt the treatment plan in an appropriate manner.

Massage Therapy and Medications represents a landmark addition to the literature available to support high quality education and professional practice by massage therapists everywhere.

John Yates, Ph.D.

Dr. John Yates received his Ph.D. from the University of Manitoba in 1976. He developed a strong interest in complementary health care education and research during a post-doctoral fellowship at the University of Calgary Faculty of Medicine, following which he joined the Division of Health Promotion and Disease Prevention in the Department of Health Care and Epidemiology at the University of British Columbia. Dr. Yates became involved with the West Coast College of Massage Therapy prior to its opening in 1983, and served as the Academic Education Director until 1997. Dr. Yates was the founding President of the Physical Medicine Research Foundation (PMRF) from 1985 to 1990, and was a member of the Medical Advisory Board of the Western Division of the PMRF from 1990 to 1993. He has also served as Research Director for the Massage Therapists' Association of B.C., is a member of the Editorial Board of the Journal of Soft Tissue Manipulation, *was instrumental in developing the curriculum standard for massage therapy in British Columbia, and is the author of* A Physician's Guide to Therapeutic Massage, *now in its second edition. Dr. Yates is currently living in Arizona and provides consulting services to accreditation and certification organizations, professional associations, and colleges of massage therapy throughout North America.*

Outline

MASSAGE THERAPY AND MEDICATIONS

Foreword 1
Outline 4
Learning Objectives 7

BASIC CONCEPTS AND GUIDELINES

Chapter 1
Why Massage Therapists Need to Know How Medications Work 11
Chapter 2
Common Pharmaceutical Terms and Concepts 15
Chapter 3
How Drugs are Administered to the Body 27
Chapter 4
Drug Processing in the Body 37
Chapter 5
General Treatment Guidelines 43
      Case History Form 48
      Letter to Health Care Practitioner 53

COMMONLY PRESCRIBED MEDICATIONS AND TREATMENT PLANNING

Chapter 6
Drugs for Managing Pain and Inflammation 79
      Non-Steroidal Anti-Inflammatory Drugs (NSAIDS) 79
      Narcotic Analgesics 81
      Skeletal Muscle Relaxants 84
      Corticosteroids 86

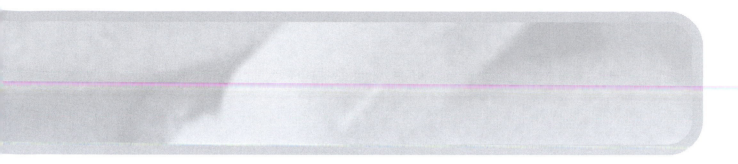

Chapter 7

Drugs for Managing Cardiovascular Disease 97
  Drugs that Improve Heart Function 101
  Drugs that Increase Blood Vessel Diameter 104
  Drugs that Alter Blood Coagulation Mechanisms .109
  Drugs that Reduce Blood Volume 113
  Drugs that Lower Blood Lipid Levels 115

Chapter 8

Drugs for Managing Diabetes Mellitus 125
  Insulin 127
  Oral Hypoglycemic Drugs 131

Chapter 9

Drugs for Managing Respiratory Inflammation and Congestion 145
  Drugs that Treat/Manage Allergic Reactions 148
  Drugs that Increase Airway Diameter 150
  Drugs that Manage Respiratory Congestion 153
  Drugs that Suppress Coughing 154

Chapter 10

Drugs for Managing Mood and Emotional Disorders .163
  Anti-Anxiety Medications 165
  Antidepressants 168
  Antipsychotic Medications 173

Chapter 11

Drugs for Managing Cancer 185
  Antineoplastic Drugs 192
  Antinausea or Anti-Emetic Drugs 199

Chapter 12

Drugs for Managing HIV/AIDS 209
  Antiviral Drugs 213

BIBLIOGRAPHY 226
INDEX 231

Learning Objectives

The information presented in this book will give the reader:

- a basic understanding of the concepts and principles of pharmacology

- familiarity with pharmacological terms

- more confidence researching drugs and reading drug profiles

- an introduction to how the body processes and utilizes medications

- an awareness of how drugs are administered and an appreciation of how different methods of administration affect massage therapy treatment

- an understanding of the importance of including medication information in your case history taking

- an appreciation of the categories of drugs that are employed in the management of a number of common disorders

- basic principles about how the mechanisms of drug action can interact with the effects of massage therapy

- an awareness of how drugs the client is taking may influence assessment results

- an understanding of how medication effects can influence selection and application of massage techniques and hydrotherapy

- an 'at your fingertips' reference to common drug side effects

- an awareness of how certain drug effects can contraindicate massage or make it necessary to postpone treatments

- some pointers about exercise recommendation related to medication effects

- more confidence in designing safe and effective treatment plans taking into account the medications the client is using

Basic
Concepts
and
Guidelines

CHAPTER 1

Why Massage Therapists Need to Know How Medications Work

When the suggestion is made that massage therapists should receive more training in one area or another, the response is often that the proposed subject is really postgraduate education. It is argued that practitioners who wish to pursue a particular interest can always elect to do more training, but the additional education is not necessary for everyday clinical practice. Whether valid or not in other contexts, this argument is not well founded when applied to massage therapists and their need for knowledge of basic pharmacology.

While some massage therapists make a definite decision to work in injury rehabilitation, palliative care, and other such medically intense settings, many say they could not have predicted at graduation the paths their practices would take. The truth is that most massage practitioners encounter an unpredictable variety of clinical conditions in their client populations. Today massage therapists are becoming more and more actively involved in the integrated health care management of some of our most challenging diseases.

On the surface of things, it is easy to underestimate a massage therapist's need to know about medications. Traditionally only members of a mainstream medical profession, like doctors, nurses, and dentists, have received instruction in pharmacology. The reality is, however, that massage therapists treat clients on a daily basis who are taking various types of prescribed drugs. In many cases these medications affect body physiology in ways that make modifying massage treatment necessary.

Clients who visit massage therapy clinics for relaxation, or seek out massage in settings like spas or fitness centers, are often taking drugs for heart problems, arthritis, cancer, diabetes, AIDS, depression, chronic pain, and so on. The fact that the focus of the treatment may be stress reduction or routine self care does not mean that the interaction between the client's medication and the massage therapy given is a non-issue. This is also true about treatment modalities that might be considered 'light' like lymphatic drainage, or more energy-focused like craniosacral therapy. Since there is a drug in the client's body, the practitioner has to have basic information about how it may impact on the client's responses to the treatment about to be given.

A standard definition of pharmacology is "the study of the action of chemicals on living organisms to produce biological effects." Pharmacology is subdivided into areas including pharmacodynamics, pharmacokinetics, pharmacy, and toxicology, all of which support the understanding and utilization of medications in medical treatment.

Massage therapy is generically defined as "the manipulation of the soft tissues of the body for a therapeutic response." In addition to direct manual manipulation of tissues, other modalities are often used during treatment. Examples include hydrotherapy, actinotherapy, and aromatherapy, as well as specific manual techniques like joint mobilization, manual lymph drainage, muscle energy techniques, and myofascial release methods. All are geared towards producing physical changes for the benefit of the client.

Both pharmacy and massage therapy, although very different disciplines, attempt to create physiologic and psychological changes important to the achievement of better health and quality of life.

All medications affect the normal responses of the body in some way. While some of these effects are not relevant to massage practice, in many cases the combined physiological results enhance or alter the impact of massage therapy modalities. At times the outcome can be adverse. For example:

- Centrally acting skeletal muscle relaxants (e.g. cyclobenzaprine) depress various parts of the central nervous system. This can alter the normal protective stretch reflexes in skeletal muscles so that there is potential for damage from manual techniques.

- The phenothiazines (e.g. trifluoperazine) are used for their anti-psychotic properties. They often alter the temperature regulating mechanisms of the body, creating an important hydrotherapy concern.

- Corticosteroids (e.g. dexamethasone) are a group of drugs widely used in medicine to control pain, inflammation, and immune responses. These drugs are also known to weaken connective tissues including skin, fascia, ligaments, and muscle.

Let's take a look at two scenarios that illustrate why a massage practitioner needs to know basic information about drug effects and interactions:

1. The massage technique of petrissage creates hyperemia, while the application of heat either locally (a hot pack) or systemically (sitting in a whirlpool or hot herbal bath) creates vasodilation. Both have the direct effect of increasing blood flow into the affected tissues. If your client is taking medications for a cardiovascular complaint, the response to such modalities may be altered due to the effects of the medication on the circulatory system. A predisposition to adverse reactions is therefore created. For example, petrissage can cause bruising in someone taking an anticoagulant, and a hot systemic treatment such as a whirlpool may promote fatigue, dizziness, and even fainting in combination with a vasodilator medication.

2. A client with a sore shoulder is taking a pain-relieving drug, such as aspirin or ibuprofen, and also seeks out massage treatment. The client requests

"deep work" to get to the root of the problem, which is a combination of tendinitis and old scar tissue. The therapist complies and gives a rigorous deep treatment. The next day the client is very bruised and in much worse pain. If the therapist had been aware that aspirin and ibuprofen have anticoagulant properties as well as reducing the ability to give accurate feedback about how painful a technique is, it would have been clear that the 'deep work' approach was not indicated at that time.

The general population is increasingly combining allopathic medicine (using drugs to treat a condition and/or alleviate symptoms) and non-drug therapies such as massage. This combining of therapies by the American public was first documented in a study published in 1993.[1] The data indicated that 83% of individuals interviewed saw both their medical doctor and providers of "unconventional" medicine[2] in their search for better health, even when they had serious medical conditions. The study additionally found that 72% did not inform their physician that they were receiving these other therapies while under medical care. Whatever the reasons for this are, it speaks to the need for practitioners of complementary health care methods to have independent awareness of the implications of combining their treatments with common allopathic modalities.

When a client reports: "My doctor has prescribed muscle relaxants for me," or "I have been taking a painkiller since the accident," or "I got a steroid shot for the bursitis," the massage therapist needs to understand the significance of these statements as they relate to massage treatment planning. The practitioner is responsible for both the effectiveness and the safety of the therapy provided.

To provide safe and effective treatment, massage therapists should have:

- a basic understanding of the actions and effects of commonly used drugs, and the ability to research the effects of other medications encountered

- knowledge of how massage affects the body's physiology and the ability to apply this knowledge to varying client presentations

It is not the intention of this text to provide extensive coverage of all drugs or detailed discussion of the chemical structures of drugs. Nor does the mention of specific drugs or brand names imply their superiority over others or constitute a recommendation for their specific use.

When therapists require specific information about a medication, there are a number of good resource texts such as *The Physicians Desk Reference (PDR)*, *The United States Pharmacopeial Drug Information (USP DI)*, and the *Compendium of Pharmaceuticals and Specialties (CPS)*, which is a Canadian reference for health care professionals. In some cases, the pharmacist or attending physician is also an important resource.

Massage therapists can feel at a loss when approaching a doctor or researching in such reference texts because the language used to discuss medications can be quite technical. It is also important to be aware that the available resources usually do not reflect an understanding of the effects of massage therapy and the impact of combining massage modalities with the drug in question.

A useful resource in understanding how massage therapy affects the body is *A Physician's Guide to Therapeutic Massage* by Dr. John Yates. This book presents research findings that discuss the physiologic effects of massage therapy on the various body systems. Research into how massage therapy influences the body physiologically is still limited and is ongoing; therapists are reminded to use the available information as a guide and to stay alert for individual client reactions.

This text is designed to help massage therapists understand the language and concepts of pharmacology and how the use of medications relates to massage therapy. It also provides information about the potential impact that drugs can have on a massage treatment and offers guidelines for preventing practitioner-induced adverse effects through appropriate planning and treatment adaptation.

1. Eisenberg, D.M., et al.,"Unconventional Medicine in the United States, Prevalence, Cost and Patterns of Use," *New England Journal of Medicine*, January 28, 1993.

2. Unconventional medicine was defined as "…medical interventions not taught widely at U.S. medical schools or generally available at U.S. hospitals. Examples include acupuncture, chiropractic, and massage therapy."

CHAPTER 2

Common Pharmaceutical Terms and Concepts

To have a clearer understanding of how drugs work therapists must be able to read and understand drug profiles or monographs. Reading a drug profile can be quite challenging because it is often difficult to understand the language of pharmacology. This chapter explains commonly used terms that therapists will encounter when reading information about drugs.

1.   DRUG NAMES

Drugs are known by either their generic name or their brand name.

Generic Name

The generic name of a drug is a simplified term that reflects the official chemical name and structure of the drug. As can be seen in the example below, the generic name diazepam is much simpler and easier to use than the chemical name of the same compound.

Generic name: diazepam

Official chemical name:

    7 chloro-1,3dihydro-1-methyl-5-phenyl-2H-1,4-benzodiazepin-2-one ($C_{16}H_{13}ClN_2O$)

Sometimes a drug may have more than one generic name. For example, acetaminophen is also known as paracetamol. In this text, the most common generic name will be used.

Brand Name

When a drug is developed, researched, tested, and produced for sale in the marketplace by a drug manufacturing company, the formulation is assigned a brand name. The brand name is the registered trademark ® for a generic drug by a drug manufacturer.

The generic drug called acetaminophen or paracetamol is more commonly known by its brand name Tylenol. Another example is the generic drug ibuprofen, which is known by several brand names including Motrin, Advil, Nuprin, and Brufen.

The use of a brand name in this book does not imply its superiority over a brand name not included, nor is it intended to be a recommendation for its use.

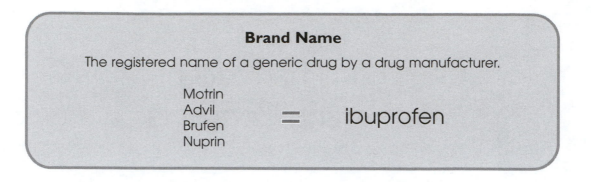

Brand Name

The registered name of a generic drug by a drug manufacturer.

Motrin
Advil   =   ibuprofen
Brufen
Nuprin

Clinical Relevance

In today's very competitive medication market an increasing number of companies are manufacturing generic drug preparations that typically sell at a cheaper price than the corresponding brand name version. Although these preparations meet official requirements, concerns about their therapeutic effectiveness and tolerability do sometimes arise when compared to their brand name counterparts. On the other hand, they can be more efficacious for some people.

You will no doubt encounter clients who have changed their medication from a brand name drug to the generic version or from a generic to the brand name. If it is a prescribed change, most likely the physician will be monitoring the client. However, it is also possible to voluntarily change a medication by obtaining a prescription from another doctor or by ordering it over the Internet. If the change is not being professionally monitored, and the client experiences adverse reactions such as dizziness, nausea, or headaches, these symptoms may not be correctly attributed to the generic/brand name drug switchover.

Another concern about this type of medication change is that the client may not experience the same degree of therapeutic effectiveness as with the version of the drug originally being taken. This can be life threatening if the client has a serious condition and is making the switch without appropriate medical supervision. It may also make reactions to massage therapy suddenly less amenable.

Massage practitioners are encouraged to be alert to clients changing medications between generic and brand name versions, and to inquire about any adverse reactions or side effects experienced since the change.

2. DRUG CLASSIFICATION

Drugs can be classified in several ways. For example, for the purposes of regulatory bodies they can be broadly classified as:

- non-prescription drugs
- prescription drugs
- restricted and controlled drugs

Drugs can also be classified according to their medicinal and chemical properties. They are often grouped according to their:

- therapeutic properties
- action or effect on a specific body system
- chemical structures

The recommendation of a specific member of a drug class by a physician depends on various factors such as cost, patient tolerance, and pharmacokinetic properties.

When a massage therapist is reading a drug profile, particular attention should be paid to the classification of drugs according to their therapeutic effects, and what body systems are most affected.

Classification by Therapeutic Effect

When drugs have been placed together in a class based on similar therapeutic properties, this is because they are generally used in the management of a particular disorder or disease. As a result, when a specific effect is needed the physician can select from a range of drugs. For example, if the desired therapeutic effect is to reduce blood pressure, the physician can prescribe either one or a combination of drugs that are known to have an antihypertensive effect. This class includes drug categories like the diuretics, beta blockers, calcium channel blockers, and vasodilators. Regardless of how they act to reduce blood pressure, these chemicals are classified as 'antihypertensive drugs.'

Let's look at another example. If the desired therapeutic effect is to reduce pain, the physician can prescribe either one or a combination of drugs that are known to have an analgesic effect. This is a large class of medications involving many categories. Examples include the non-steroidal anti-inflammatory drugs, the narcotic analgesics, and the centrally acting skeletal muscle relaxants.

Classification by Effect on a Specific Body System

When drugs are classified according to their body system effects, their placement in a class does not necessarily reflect what their therapeutic use might be. For example, drugs that affect the central nervous system (CNS) include the CNS stimulants, such as caffeine, and CNS depressants like the narcotic analgesics. Drugs that affect the function of the gastrointestinal tract include the antacids, which are used to neutralize stomach acidity; laxatives, used for the management of constipation; and antidiarrheal drugs for the management of diarrhea.

Classification by Chemical Structure

When drugs are classified according to their chemical structure they often show related therapeutic properties. Slight changes in chemical structure can create drugs with weaker or stronger therapeutic effects and different side effects. This can be observed in the range of medications included in large groupings like the corticosteroids, narcotics, beta blockers, and non-steroidal anti-inflammatories.

Clinical Relevance

A client may not remember the name of the medication(s) he or she is taking, but will be able to tell you the reason it was prescribed, for example to lower blood pressure. Until more specific information is provided by the client, knowledge of this systemic drug classification should guide you toward planning an appropriate assessment and treatment that pays attention to the cardiovascular system problem.

Clients may also not fully comprehend why a specific drug has been prescribed, for example for back pain. Regardless of the exact cause of pain, which is a subject the massage therapist will want to explore further, the fact that the client is taking an analgesic always necessitates having an awareness of analgesic-related concerns, like reduced accuracy of client feedback.

3.   USES OR INDICATIONS

The section of a drug profile called "Uses" or "Indications" lists the diseases or disorders for which the drug is officially recommended. These are the uses approved by the Food and Drug Administration (FDA) or similar Health and Welfare department of the country of origin.

Sometimes drugs are employed in an unofficial or experimental manner. An illustration of this is the current recommendation of aspirin in cardiovascular disease. The official use for aspirin is the management of mild to moderate pain. However, because of its anticoagulant effects aspirin is now being widely recommended to help prevent heart attacks and strokes. It is also showing very promising results when used in the treatment and management of certain types of colon cancer.

Information about non-official uses of medications can usually be obtained through sources like the local library or pharmacist, the Internet, or a medical health care provider.

As more research and testing is conducted, a once experimental use of a drug may receive regulatory body approval and become an official use.

Clinical Relevance

A single medication can have several approved and non-approved uses. Therapists should always inquire about why a client is taking a particular medication. Looking at the range of uses for aspirin given on the next page, you can see that the reason a client is taking it is important to discern, as the approach to assessment and treatment for a headache will be quite different than that for treating an inflamed joint.

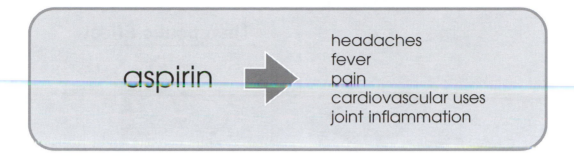

aspirin → headaches
fever
pain
cardiovascular uses
joint inflammation

4.   EFFECTS OF MEDICATIONS

The effects of medications can be grouped into three categories:

- therapeutic effects
- side effects or adverse effects
- unpredictable effects

Drug effects are influenced by factors such as dosage, age and gender of the patient, lifestyle, pathologies present, and the person's own unique constitution.

Therapeutic Effect

The therapeutic effect is the desired effect of the drug. For example, a therapeutic effect of aspirin is to reduce the pain and inflammation of arthritis, and the therapeutic effect of the anti-anxiety drug diazepam is to calm and relax the user. The therapeutic effect of a drug is intended to help the user get better.

Side Effect

Also referred to as adverse effects, side effects are the undesirable reactions a drug can produce. They may be related to the therapeutic effect of the drug, being in essence a stronger than typically experienced response. For example, in some individuals diazepam can promote a greater degree of calming and relaxation than desired. The result may be drowsiness to an extent where the ability to drive or operate machinery is impaired.

Side effects can also be the result of additional actions a drug may have. Aspirin, aside from its desired therapeutic effects, irritates the lining of the stomach. This irritation can lead to the development of gastric ulcers and even severe gastrointestinal bleeding.

Side effects may also be created by interactions among two or more medications. In other words, two drugs that individually may not produce problematic responses, when combined, can result in new or intensified adverse effects.

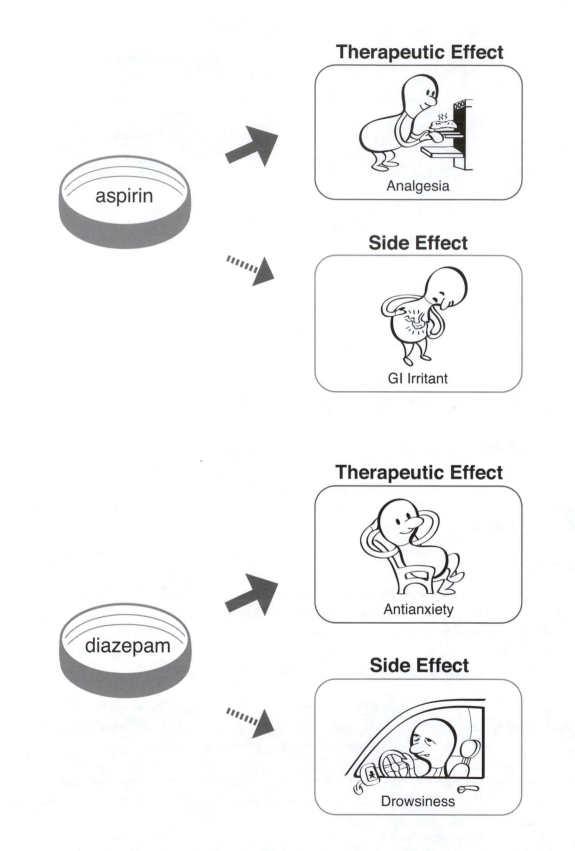

Therapeutic Effect

aspirin

Analgesia

Side Effect

GI Irritant

Therapeutic Effect

diazepam

Antianxiety

Side Effect

Drowsiness

Side effects may be caused by additional actions of a drug, for example aspirin irritating the stomach lining, or an intensification of a drug's actions, as in the case of valium producing drowsiness.

Unpredictable Effect

Unpredictable effects of a drug tend to occur in two types:

- allergic or hypersensitivity reactions
- idiosyncratic reactions

Allergic or Hypersensitivity Reactions

Some people react allergically to some drugs. These types of reactions can range from fairly mild to quite severe. Mild reactions usually manifest as skin eruptions such as hives. Other mild allergic reactions to drugs can include joint pain, fever, and swollen lymph nodes.

If the allergic response is more severe, the client can experience an anaphylaxis reaction or anaphylactic shock. Anaphylaxis is a medical emergency situation characterized by seriously decreased blood pressure and restricted airflow, the latter being a result of contraction of the bronchial smooth muscle and swelling of the throat and mouth.

Idiosyncratic Reactions

Idiosyncratic reactions are unexpected or highly unusual effects of a medication, occurring uniquely in individuals or in very small numbers of people. This type of effect can be difficult to explain, although genetic predisposition may play a role. When compared to the expected therapeutic response or typical side effects of the drug, idiosyncratic reactions can be accelerated, toxic, or opposite effect responses.

Clinical Relevance

Clients can be experiencing effects from their medications other than the desired therapeutic ones. In some cases a client's chief complaint may actually be a drug side effect. Therapists are encouraged to always check with clients concerning what side effects they have experienced, and/or what they have been told may occur. Common side effects are usually listed in drug profiles. In a later section of this book, side effect tables are presented for the drug classes commonly seen in massage therapy practice. It is important to keep in mind that such lists can never be considered exhaustive given the range of responses to medications that may occur.

Practitioners should always monitor client symptomatology and be alert for unusual aspects, unexpected changes, or atypical responses to massage treatment modalities. If adverse or unpredictable drug effects are suspected, the client should be advised to schedule a follow-up session with the prescribing medical practitioner.

When clients are taking more than one medication there is an increased likelihood that the combination of drug effects may result in side effects or idiosyncratic reactions, some of which may contribute to their musculoskeletal and general health complaints.

5. MECHANISM OF ACTION

This term describes what a drug does inside the body to produce its therapeutic effect(s). Drugs do not create new functions; instead they alter existing cellular activities. The processes through which medications influence body physiology are varied and often biochemically complex. With some drugs these biochemical reactions are well researched and documented, while for others the exact processes and mechanisms involved are not fully understood, or not known.

Drug mechanisms of action are created through one or a combination of the following:

• By Combining with Specific Cellular Receptors

In order for a drug to exert its biological effect there must be an interaction between the drug molecules and the target cells. The "lock and key" theory postulated in 1894 by Emil Fischer, a German chemist and enzymologist, offers an explanation as follows: All cells have receptor sites on their membranes that will only fit with molecules of a certain size, shape, or charge (+ve or -ve). When a drug molecule is a good match with a cell membrane's receptor sites, it can produce changes inside the cell such as altering internal ion channels, messenger systems, or enzyme reactions. These changes adjust how the cell functions in order to create the drug's effects. The interaction between the drug molecule and the cell membrane is compared to the fit between a lock (cell) and key (drug molecule).

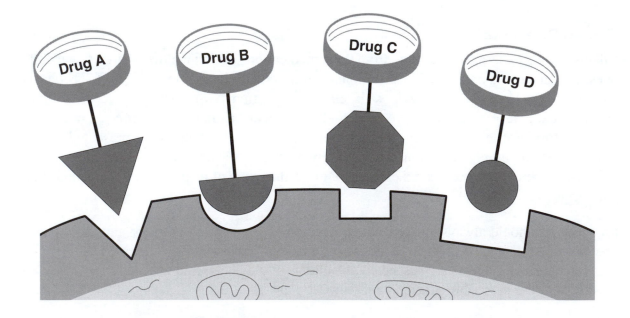

Lock and key configuration between drug and cell receptor: Drugs A and B each fit into a matching receptor on the cell surface and will therefore be able to alter the cell's functions. Drugs C and D do not have matching shapes and will not have any impact on the cell.

To give some clinical examples:

1. A drug may interact with a muscle cell receptor site to cause prolonged opening of an internal calcium channel. This results in increased calcium utilization in the cell and produces the drug's effect, which in this instance is an increase in the force of muscle contraction. Such an effect can be useful in supporting a weakened heart, for example.

2. If the mechanism of action of a drug is to increase the sensitivity of cell membranes to insulin, the result being to decrease blood glucose levels, the drug is useful in the management of Type II diabetes.

• By Chemically Altering Body Fluids

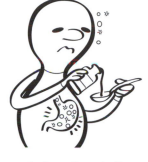

A common example of this mechanism of action is taking an antacid to neutralize excess stomach acidity and reduce or prevent digestive discomfort.

• By Chemically Altering Cell Membranes

Drugs can act on a cell's membrane to alter its electrical stability and therefore influence its responsiveness to stimuli. Typically, the drug will influence the membrane's permeability, causing speeding up or slowing down of the movement of ions into and out of the cell. Some examples of medications that act this way include lithium and the general anaesthetic gases.

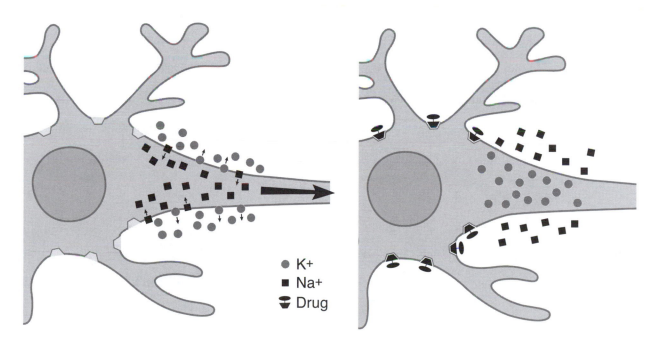

This neuron is being influenced by a medication to be less easily depolarized. This effect is desirable in a number of circumstances, for example to produce local anaesthesia or prevent seizures.

• By Interacting with Extracellular Enzyme Systems

Enzymes are protein molecules that facilitate or catalyse all chemical reactions of living cells, causing them to respond in various ways. By influencing enzyme behaviors, medications can have numerous types of impacts on tissue function.

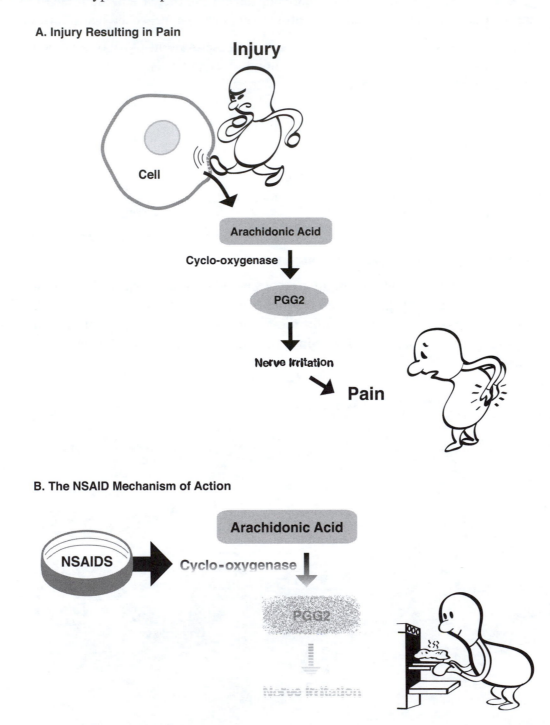

A. Injury Resulting in Pain

Injury

Cell

Arachidonic Acid

Cyclo-oxygenase

PGG2

Nerve Irritation

Pain

B. The NSAID Mechanism of Action

NSAIDS

Arachidonic Acid

Cyclo-oxygenase

PGG2

Nerve Irritation

Illustration of how aspirin and other non-steroidal anti-inflammatory drugs reduce pain by blocking the activity of the cyclooxygenase enzyme, resulting in inhibition of prostaglandin synthesis.

Clinical Relevance

Knowledge of the mechanism of action of a drug increases one's understanding of why the drug is being used for a particular condition or conditions, and why the drug produces its effects. More importantly, it is often the basis for the practitioner's awareness of how massage therapy might promote intensified or adverse reactions. Alternatively, it may explain why massage therapy will have limited effectiveness while the drug is being taken. Numerous examples of how drug mechanisms of action can influence the impact of massage modalities will be discussed in later sections of this book.

6. HALF-LIFE

Half-life in the pharmaceutical context is the time it takes for the body's normal metabolic and elimination processes to reduce the blood concentration of the drug to one half, or 50%. For example, if there is 100 mg of a medication in the bloodstream, the half-life of the drug is the time it would take to reduce its blood concentration to 50 mg. Each drug has its own individual half-life.

Assuming a half-life of 20 minutes, the table that follows illustrates how much of the drug mentioned above would be in the bloodstream after 100 minutes.

TIME IN MINUTES	BLOOD CONCENTRATION (mg)
start amount	100
20	50
40	25
60	12.5
80	6.25
100	3.125

Clinical Relevance

There are many biochemical processes involved in the metabolism and elimination of drugs from the body. The kidneys and liver are key organs in these processes. Clients who have dysfunction of either of these organs may be especially vulnerable to adverse and toxic reactions because of ineffective removal of drugs and their metabolites. Therapists are encouraged to inquire about the health and function of these organs and be alert to the potential implications of dysfunction.

7. ONSET OF ACTION

This term refers to the time it takes before the user feels the effects of the drug. The key factor is usually how the drug was administered. For example, the onset of action can be felt almost immediately following an intravenous injection, but most solid orally administered preparations take about half an hour. Some drugs require concentration accumulation in target body parts. An example of this is the accumulation of an anti-inflammatory medication within the synovial joint, which can involve several days before peak onset of action is experienced.

Clinical Relevance

Knowing the expected onset of action of a drug can help the practitioner determine optimal scheduling of massage therapy. Wherever possible, appointments should be planned when the effect of the medication is most conducive to safe and effective treatment. In some cases, this will be when the drug is exercising maximum effect and in others when it is not. Guidelines elaborating these relationships will be offered in a later chapter. Therapists are expected to exercise professional judgement, and to consult with the appropriate health care provider when necessary.

8.   BIOAVAILABILITY

The term bioavailability describes the amount of a drug that actually enters the systemic circulation and is available to produce its effects. A key factor affecting bioavailability is how the drug has been administered into the body (the route of administration). For example, if 50 mg of a drug is taken orally but the amount that actually reaches the circulation, due to the impact of digestive processes, is 25 mg, the drug has a 50% bioavailability. If, however, 50 mg of the drug is administered directly into the bloodstream via intravenous injection, it is 100% bioavailable.

When a medication has a low bioavailability only a small quantity of the drug is available in the blood. Most of the administered dose is either changed into another form or excreted before it enters the bloodstream. On the other hand, drugs with high bioavailability have high available concentrations in the systemic circulation and are usually rapidly absorbed after administration.

Other factors that influence drug bioavailability include dosage and frequency and the person's age and general health. The presence of any pathologies that affect how the drug is absorbed, for example gastrointestinal disorders if the drug is administered orally, will also play a role.

Clinical Relevance

Like onset of action, bioavailability can be a factor in massage treatment scheduling and design. Having information about a medication's bioavailability adds to the elements the massage therapist brings together to create a safe and appropriate treatment plan. For example, if the client is being massaged in hospital and is receiving an analgesic medication via IV, the impact of the drug will be consistently strong and the massage therapist will need to take into account the client's inability to give trustworthy feedback about depth of technique. On the other hand, when a client is taking an analgesic orally, treatment can be organized around whether the maximum analgesic effect is helpful (e.g. in palliative care) or of concern, for example when frictioning a tendinitis.

CHAPTER 3

How Drugs are Administered to the Body

"Route of administration" is the term used to describe how a drug is administered to the body. Drugs can be administered to a specific body area for a local effect or they can be applied in a manner that has a systemic effect.

The routes of administration discussed in this chapter include:

- oral (into the gastrointestinal tract in solid or liquid form)
- mucous membrane application (under the tongue, inhaled, rectal)
- topical (application to the ears, eyes, skin)
- parenteral (by injection)
- implanted catheters and drug pumps

The route of administration influences the rate and completeness of absorption of the drug into the bloodstream. This in turn affects several pharmacologic properties of the drug, including its bioavailability, onset, and intensity of action. Knowledge of routes of administration will have an impact on the timing and design of the massage treatment, as will be discussed later.

1.   ORAL ADMINISTRATION

The oral route of administration is by far the most popular way of introducing drugs into the body. The medication is swallowed in the prescribed dose and absorption occurs into the blood from the gastrointestinal tract. Solid oral preparations include tablets, caplets, and capsules; liquid preparations include syrups, elixirs, and suspensions. Depending on the form of oral administration (liquid or solid) it usually takes between a few minutes and an hour before the drug is absorbed and distributed in the bloodstream and the person begins to experience its effects. The maximum effect occurs when a peak level is achieved in the blood.

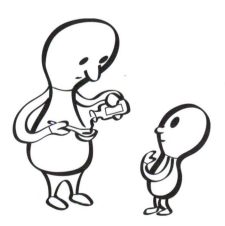

Solid preparations will typically dissolve in the stomach and be absorbed into the blood from the intestines a half to one hour after administration. Enteric coated and timed release preparations are an exception to this. Enteric coated tablets/caplets have a specially designed layer of material that dissolves in the intestines instead of the stomach, sparing the stomach from direct exposure to the drug. Drugs that irritate the stomach lining, such as aspirin and other non-steroidal anti-inflammatory drugs (NSAIDs), usually have an enteric coat. Enteric coated drugs may take a slightly longer time to be absorbed into the bloodstream, and the onset of action of these preparations can depend on several factors including whether or not there is food in the stomach, and how fast the stomach empties.

Timed release preparations are also referred to as "controlled release" or "slow release." Following oral administration only a certain amount or part of the preparation will become available for absorption into the blood. The remaining parts will dissolve at later times as the preparation passes through the intestines. This property of dissolving at different times ensures a constant level of medication in the blood. Timed release preparations are usually administered once or twice a day.

Liquid medications are generally absorbed into the circulation within 15 minutes after oral administration and usually have a faster onset of action when compared to the solid oral preparations.

2. APPLICATION TO MUCOUS MEMBRANES

Mucous membranes contain mucus-secreting cells and cover the internal surfaces of body passages. The digestive, respiratory, reproductive, and urinary tracts are all lined by mucous membranes.

Mucous membranes are highly vascularized. They have extensive networks of blood vessels that tend to pose fewer restrictions to drug access than the skin or intestinal cells. Local applications are used to address infections and inflammations, for example a canker sore in the mouth, but their vascularization also makes mucous membranes a good route of administration when a systemic effect with a more rapid onset of action is needed.

A common example of a systemic use in a situation that requires quick action is the management of angina attacks. At the beginning of the attack the client places a nitroglycerine tablet under his or her tongue (sublingual administration). The tablet dissolves and is absorbed across the mucous membrane

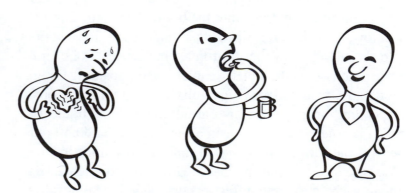

of the oral cavity directly into the bloodstream. Its symptom relieving effect on the heart occurs within minutes.

Drugs are applied to mucous membranes as:

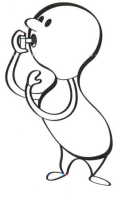

- suppositories or enemas applied into the rectum
- inhalations in powder, gas, dust, or vapour forms that are usually administered into the respiratory tract from specialized devices
- sprays and drops applied into the oral and respiratory tracts
- swabs, powders, sublingual and buccal (dissolved in the cheek pouch) tablets applied into the mouth and throat
- douches, foams, creams, and pessaries (vaginal suppositories) applied into the vagina

3.   TOPICAL APPLICATIONS

Topical applications are preparations applied:

- into the ear (otic)
- into the eye (ophthalmic)
- onto the skin (dermal)

They are generally used to treat local complaints such as ear infections, eye irritations, and itchy skin.

Otic Administration

Medications are usually administered into the ear as drops. The drops are applied as close to body temperature as possible to avoid overstimulation of the auditory nerve. Occasionally clients may experience vertigo type symptoms. Often a piece of dry cotton will be inserted into the ear after application to absorb any excess medication.

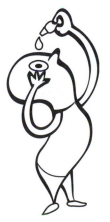

Ophthalmic Administration

Drops or ointments are the usual way of administering drugs into the eye. The preparations must be kept as sterile as possible because the eyes are very susceptible to infection. Administration of eye medications may be followed by periods of blurred vision.

Dermal Administration

Dermal applications are becoming a more and more popular way of administering medications. They are used in several ways, including:

- to treat local skin conditions such as rashes, dry skin, infections, and abrasions

- for the relief of muscle and joint pain

- for the systemic administration of drugs

The skin, which is the largest organ of the body, has many functions. It is waterproof; it protects against invasion of microorganisms; and it acts as a barrier to ultraviolet radiation. Under normal conditions the skin also acts as a barrier to most chemicals. However, because of differences in thickness (e.g. thin behind the ears and in the inner upper forearm, thick on the palm of the hand and sole of the foot), and the penetrating nature of certain chemicals, the ability of substances to penetrate the dermal boundary varies. Chemicals that are able to cross the skin's barriers and enter the circulation will have a systemic effect on the body.

Drugs are applied to the skin as ointments, creams, gels, solutions, and more recently as the skin patch.

Topical Skin Applications for Local Use

Topical applications of creams, ointments, gels, and lotions are used to treat local skin conditions like cuts and rashes. They tend to contain ingredients such as antibiotics, antihistamines, corticosteroids, moisturizers, and analgesics. These preparations are designed to act specifically on the affected area. They are not intended to enter the systemic circulation; any such absorption that does occur is usually minute and of little concern.

Topical Skin Applications for Relief of Muscle and Joint Pain

Creams, ointments, liniments, and certain types of medicated plasters are regularly used for the relief of low-grade muscle and joint pain. Sometimes referred to as counter-irritants, they contain ingredients such as capsaicin, menthol, wintergreen, and various types of essential and medicinal oils that are quite volatile, meaning that they evaporate quickly. The exact action of each ingredient will differ, but they all affect the local circulation and superficial nerves in ways that can relieve pain and stiffness. Primarily, they tend to cause an increase in local blood flow that improves oxygen and nutrient delivery and removes metabolic wastes from the affected tissues.

When such a counter-irritant is applied, especially if it contains a medicinal oil in high concentration, the person may experience an initial coolness followed by a sensation of warmth. When this happens the oil applied to the skin surface has absorbed body heat causing it to evaporate from the skin, hence the coolness at first, and the warmth that follows represents an increase in blood flow into the area of application.

Topical Skin Applications for Systemic Administration of Drugs

Specially formulated ointments, and products like the skin patch, are increasingly becoming popular routes for the systemic administration of medications. The preparations involved are 'transdermal,' meaning that the drug is formulated in a special gel-like matrix that is able to pass through the skin barrier and enter the systemic circulation. Nicotine and hormone replacement therapy patches are common examples of this type of application. They are stuck onto the skin in much the same way we apply a Band-Aid.

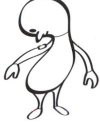

Drugs like nitroglycerine are also available in special ointment formulations for transdermal absorption. A prescribed amount of the ointment is squeezed onto a strip that is then applied securely to the patient's skin at a chosen site. The medication is absorbed in a slow steady way to ensure a good concentration in the bloodstream over a period of time.

Therapists should remember that transdermal preparations do cross the skin barrier and must not be confused with the regular local ointments and creams described earlier. While a practitioner should always take precautions against removing a dermal preparation, when the application is being used to maintain a controlled medication level in the blood the implications of wiping it off or disengaging a patch are more serious. The practitioner can also be 'dosed' by the medication if it comes in contact with his or her skin.

4.   PARENTERAL ADMINISTRATION

The term parenteral refers to any route of administration other than the oral or gastrointestinal routes. In common usage, however, this term is closely associated with injections and that is how it will be interpreted in this text.

Situations in which the parenteral route of administration is selected include:

- when oral administration would be ineffective; for example, insulin is usually delivered by injection because if taken orally it is destroyed in the stomach

- during emergency situations where a very rapid physiologic response is needed, e.g. to prevent an anaphylactic reaction following an insect bite

- for continuous provision of a steady supply of a drug via intravenous drip, usually in a medical setting like a hospital or hospice

- when a patient is vomiting and cannot take medication orally

- for administering vaccines

- when a preparation is being injected directly into a tissue, for example into an osteoarthritic joint (intra-articular injection)

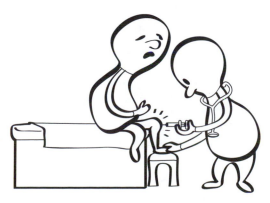

The table that follows lists routes of administration for injections, time frames for their onsets of action, and common sites of administration.

Route of Injection	Onset of Action	Site of Administration
intradermal – within the dermis of the skin	within a few minutes	often in the forearm (e.g. allergy testing), or where needed for local anaesthesia
subcutaneous – within the subcutaneous layer of the skin	can be quick, within a few minutes if there is good vascular supply	outer surface of the upper arm, the abdomen, the anterior thigh
intramuscular – within the muscle	very quick to within a few minutes; some are prepared in slow release form	the middle deltoids, the ventrogluteal area, dorsogluteal: in the region of gluteus medius or gluteus maximus, in the vastus lateralis, in the middle third of the thigh between the greater trochanter and the knee
intra-articular – directly into a joint	may take up to several hours before full effect is felt; occasionally the person may experience a flare up after the injection sometimes administered in slow release or long acting form ; effects from one injection can last up to 6 weeks	joints of the body, most commonly: shoulder, elbow, wrist, hand, hip, intervertebral, pelvis, knee, ankle, foot, sacroiliac joints
intravenous – directly into a vein	very quick to within a few minutes	median cubital, cephalic, median, and basilic veins of the elbow, forearm and dorsum of the hand
intra-arterial – directly into an artery	very quick to within a few minutes	use is restricted to special cases such as diagnostic procedures, or during chemotherapy
intrathecal – directly into the spinal column	very quick to within a few minutes	common example is the epidural (lower body anaesthesia)
intralesional – directly into a lesion	very quick to within a few minutes	for example, into trigger points or tumours
perineural (nerve block) – in the immediate vicinity of a nerve	usually within a few minutes	close to nerves, at nerve roots, in facet joints

Massage Therapy & Medications

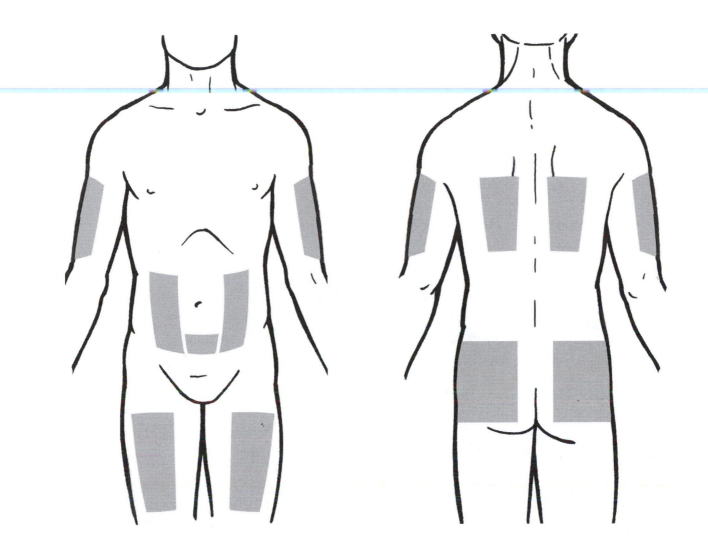

Commonly used injection sites. All sites indicated with the exception of the buttocks are frequently used for subcutaneous injections. The muscles most commonly utilized for intramuscular injections are the deltoids, the gluteals, and the quadriceps.

When a prolonged medication effect is needed, a specially prepared long-acting formulation called a **depot** (*Fr: storage*) is used. Drugs are administered in this manner by intramuscular, intra-articular, and subcutaneous injection. For example, when a person with osteoarthritis is given intra-articular injections of corticosteroids, depending on the type of corticosteroid used, the effect of the drug can last for as long as six weeks.

Some drug depot preparations are also implanted subcutaneously, for example contraceptives. The drug is slowly released and absorbed into the bloodstream. This type of contraceptive can last for up to five years.

5.   IMPLANTED CATHETERS AND DRUG PUMPS

Drug pumps and implanted catheters are another means of delivering drugs into the body. These devices are often used with patients with special requirements, for example for:

- frequent blood sample taking

- delivering many injections into the bloodstream

- giving several types of transfusions

- supplying ongoing nutritional support

- providing greater control over the administration of their medication

Implanted Catheters

An implanted catheter device is surgically fitted so that most of it is lying beneath the skin. There are two incisions made during the implantation, for entrance and exit sites. The exit site is the location where the catheter exits through the skin surface. A small length of catheter fitted with an injection cap extends beyond the exit site.

The entrance site is made in the tissue at the location where the drug is to be administered. Depending on what the medication is, and where it has to be delivered, the placement of the catheter varies. For example, if what is required is an epidural for analgesia, the catheter's entrance site is implanted into the epidural space, and if the catheter is being used to deliver insulin, the entrance site is in the subcutaneous tissues.

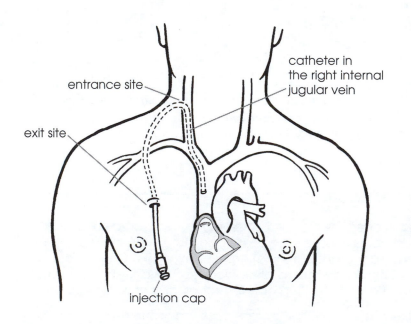

entrance site

catheter in the right internal jugular vein

exit site

injection cap

When the drug must be delivered directly into the circulation, the catheter is usually placed into a central vein. This is known as a central venous catheter (CVC). The entrance site portion is implanted with its tip threaded into a large vein, providing easy access to the vascular system without having to put a needle into a blood vessel every time a procedure is performed. The veins usually used are the large cervical veins.

The part of the catheter between the entrance and exit sites lies within a surgically created subcutaneous tunnel. An injection cap (the visible piece) is attached to the catheter at the exit site. This is the mechanism through which a needle is inserted to deliver medications.

For CVCs, the exit site of the catheter is usually on the anterior chest wall, and for epidurals on the anterior lateral flank area.

Drug Pumps

Drug pumps are sometimes used to deliver medications into the bloodstream via an intravenous line or an implanted catheter. They are 'pushing' devices in the form of an external machine or a subcutaneously implanted apparatus. With both types of pumps patients have a certain amount of control over administering their own medication.

In the external pump set-up the drug to be administered is stored inside the pump. The patient pushes a button on the pump mechanism to release a predetermined dose of the medication into the bloodstream. The pump usually regulates the intervals at which the drug can be taken to avoid overdose.

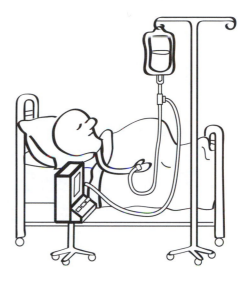

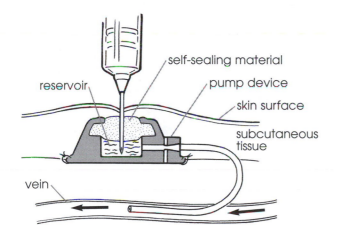

Internal pumps are subcutaneously implanted and can stay in place for as long as 1 to 2 years. Medications are injected through the skin surface into a reservoir within the pump. The patient controls the release of the medication by activating the pump with an external device much like a TV remote control. Once released the drug travels through a catheter that begins at the reservoir and terminates in a central vein.

Clinical Relevance

Knowledge of routes of administration and their implications is very useful in planning massage treatments to minimize the chances of inducing medication-related adverse reactions. For example, a client who is on short term use of oral anti-inflammatory tablets will probably give more accurate feedback about depth of technique during the treatment if it is performed when the drug's bioavailability is at its lower levels. Giving the treatment before or just after scheduled doses might be appropriate. On the other hand, when treating an insulin dependent diabetic, the medical stability of the client is of primary importance. Scheduling treatments in time periods following insulin injections so that the medication is at peak bioavailability is less likely to destabilize the diabetic condition.

Implanted catheters and drug pumps must be properly maintained by the patient and carefully monitored medically. Everyone involved with the client's care needs to maintain an awareness that infections and blood clots can develop at the entry and exit sites. A more serious concern with internally implanted drug pumps is malfunction of the pump or a blockage or kink in the delivery catheter. Such disruptions can lead to symptoms of over or under dosage of the drug.

There are a number of massage treatment guidelines that stem from specific aspects of the various routes of administration. These will be elaborated in Chapter 5.

CHAPTER 4
Drug Processing in the Body

In this chapter we will discuss what happens to a drug after it is administered into the body. Although there are differences that stem from individual drug characteristics and variations based on routes of administration, all drugs are subjected to various physiological processes that can modify their capacity to affect their target cells. These include:

- dissolving and dissociating; making the drug particles available for absorption from the gastrointestinal tract

- metabolism; processes that can change the chemical nature and activity of the drug

- distribution; delivery of the drug to its site(s) of action

- elimination; removal of the drug and its metabolites from the body

These processes have the potential to impact significantly on the therapeutic activities of drugs and properties such as their bioavailability.

1.   DISSOLVING AND DISSOCIATING

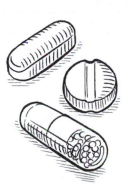

During the manufacture of solid oral medications (e.g. tablets, caplets, capsules) several inactive substances called excipients are included in the preparations. They are present in varying amounts and serve two main functions: to help the preparation maintain its stability while stored on the pharmacy shelf, and to ensure that it can readily dissolve and dissociate in the gastrointestinal tract. In the latter case they facilitate the 'breaking up' of the preparation into much smaller particles suitable for movement from the GI tract into the bloodstream. Tablets and capsules that quickly dissolve and dissociate are more rapidly absorbed. This increases the drug's bioavailability and tends to make the onset of action faster.

Orally administered liquid preparations generally contain their drug ingredients in a dissolved form, making them readily available for absorption.

Absorption of a drug into the blood is influenced by many factors. Some of these include:

- its chemical nature; for example aspirin, a weak acid, is more readily absorbed from the acidic environment of the stomach, while griseofulvin, an anti-fungal agent, is best absorbed when taken with a fatty meal

- its dosage; higher drug dosages are typically absorbed more rapidly

- its form of administration (see Chapter 3)

- the size of its particles; for example griseofulvin ultramicrosize tablets are absorbed more readily than griseofulvin microsized tablets

- the presence of any gastrointestinal pathologies (ulcers, gastritis, etc.) that can affect the amount and quality of absorption

2.   METABOLISM

Following oral administration and absorption from the intestines, a drug is transported to the liver via the portal circulation. The liver is the most important organ of metabolism. Drug profiles often contain statements such as "This drug undergoes rapid hepatic biotransformation," or "This drug is extensively metabolized by the liver." Metabolism involves a number of complex biotransformational processes which change potentially damaging substances into ones that will not be harmful to body tissues.

An aspect of metabolism that can affect drug bioavailability is called the "first pass effect." This term refers to the effects of liver processes on a drug that has just entered the blood from the GI tract. Before it can access the rest of the body via the general circulation, it is exposed to the actions of the liver's metabolizing enzymes. However, not all drugs are affected by these processes in the liver. A drug can be unaffected by metabolism, in which case it is usually excreted or eliminated in its original form.

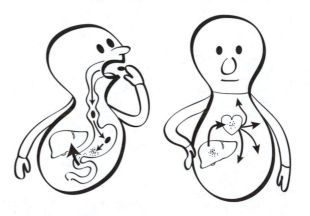

When a drug does undergo metabolism, substances called metabolites are formed. Most drug metabolites are inactive and harmless compounds, but some show various degrees of pharmacological activity. These metabolites may produce desired therapeutic effects or they may be responsible for undesired side effects. For example, describing the pharmacology of the anti-anxiety drug ketazolam, one reference text states: "The main half life of ketazolam is approximately 2 hours while half-lives of its metabolites are much longer (32-52 hours) … The main active metabolites are diazepam, …[1]" In this example both the drug and its metabolites demonstrate pharmacologic activity and produce anti-anxiety effects.

Although the liver is the key organ of metabolism, other body tissues are also involved. They include the lungs, skin, kidneys, and gastrointestinal tract. Certain enzymes found in the blood, and in neurons, are also responsible for metabolizing drugs.

Sometimes other routes of administration are used to make a drug available to its target tissues before breakdown can occur in the liver, in other words to bypass the first pass effect. For example, with sublingual administration a drug can be absorbed into the circulation through the buccal mucous membranes. From there it is transported by the superior vena cava to the heart and distributed throughout the body. Similarly, with suppository application a medication can be absorbed through the rectal mucous membranes into the circulation and enter the heart via the inferior vena cava. In both examples the heart initially distributes the drug systemically, allowing it to reach its target cells before it is taken to the liver. Intravenous or intramuscular injections are also routes of administration that allow a drug to avoid the first pass effect. By entering the systemic circulation before contacting the liver, a medication's bioavailability can be maximized and its effects experienced within a few minutes. In the normal course of blood circulation it will eventually be taken to the liver and exposed to its enzymes, at which point its bioavailability will go down.

When a systemic effect is needed very quickly, and a parenteral route is not appropriate, the sublingual route is most often employed. The example of sublingual nitroglycerine use at the onset of angina pains has already been mentioned. The resulting therapeutic effect occurs within minutes. If the nitroglycerine were taken as a swallowed tablet, the processes it would have to undergo in the gastrointestinal tract and the liver would greatly reduce its bioavailability, the timeliness of its onset of action, and its therapeutic effect.

3.   DISTRIBUTION

This term refers to how a drug is transported from its site of absorption to its site(s) of action, metabolism, and excretion. There are many complex pharmacologic and physiologic factors that support the distribution of drugs throughout the body. The ones discussed below provide a general overview of circulatory factors that can affect drug distribution.

• The Rate of Blood (and Therefore Drug) Flow to the Various Tissues

Because tissues like the kidneys, liver, and brain (for drugs that cross the blood brain barrier) consistently receive high volumes of blood, they will initially receive higher drug concentrations than do tissues like fat and muscles. As the drug is subsequently recirculated through the body, more even distribution will occur.

• How Much Drug is Bound to Plasma Proteins

Drugs in the bloodstream are often 'bound' to plasma proteins (mainly albumin) to form drug-protein complexes. Each drug has its characteristic degree of plasma protein binding.

For example, if a drug is described as 60% bound to plasma proteins this means that at any given time only 40% of the drug is 'free' in the blood to diffuse to the target tissues and cause cellular reactions. Regardless of the drug concentration, 60% will always be plasma protein bound and only 40% free in the blood.

This binding of drugs to albumin is reversible. There is constant movement of drug molecules from the bloodstream into the intercellular spaces, and reformation of new drug-protein complexes within the blood. Throughout these processes a drug's characteristic equilibrium between protein bound and free drug concentrations is maintained. Drugs that are typically highly bound to plasma proteins tend to remain in the body longer than drugs that are less so.

• Mechanisms that Control Brain Access

The blood brain barrier (BBB) consists of tightly packed endothelial cells and surrounding astrocytes which, among other things, help protect brain tissue from potentially harmful effects of drugs. How they perform their function is not fully understood, but they appear to identify substances that are potentially damaging and obstruct them from leaving the blood to enter the brain interstitium.

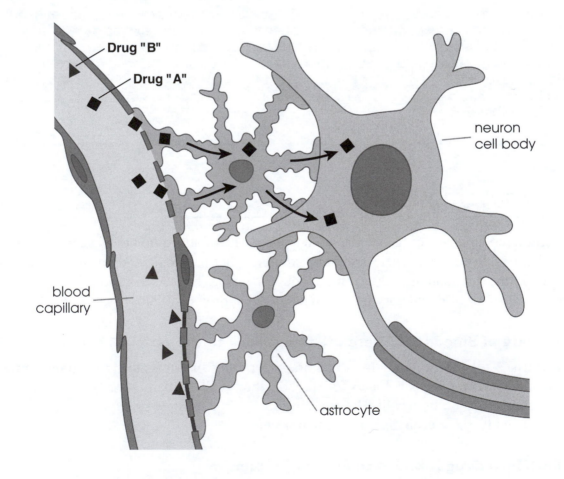

Drug A is being permitted to pass through the capillary wall and the astrocyte to gain access to the neuron; Drug B is not being allowed past the 'blood brain barrier.'

The solubility of a drug also appears to be a determining factor in whether it will gain access to the brain. Lipid soluble drugs such as the barbiturates cross the blood brain barrier much more easily than drugs with poor lipid solubility like the penicillin antibiotics.

Research also seems to suggest that a specific set of transport mechanisms are in place that influence which substances will gain access into the brain. For example glucose, which is necessary for neuron function and is water rather than lipid soluble, is transported into brain tissue dissolved in plasma.

4.   ELIMINATION

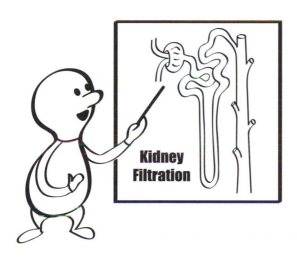

Kidney Filtration

Drugs and other toxic substances are prepared for elimination from the body by various metabolic processes in the liver. The metabolites are biochemically altered to make them harmless to body tissues and more readily eliminated.

The kidneys are the main organs involved in elimination; however, other routes include the sweat glands, bile, bowels, lungs, and even mother's milk. Drug monographs will include statements like "60% of the dose was excreted in the urine with the remaining drug undergoing fecal excretion."

Clinical Relevance

In Chapter 2, differences between generic and brand name drugs were discussed and the suggestion was made that clients who change their medication from one to another may experience adverse reactions or altered therapeutic effects. This chapter should shed more light on this issue. During the production of solid oral preparations such as tablets and capsules, the quality of excipients or inactive substances used by manufacturers varies. Since these excipients play an important role in facilitating dissolving and dissociating of the drug in the gastric environment, a tablet that dissolves and dissociates poorly will not be absorbed as readily as a tablet of higher quality. Less absorption of the drug into the bloodstream leads to lower bioavailability, slower onset of action, and questionable therapeutic effectiveness.

Clients with gastrointestinal disturbances such as vomiting and diarrhea, or who have GI disorders like ulcers or Crohn's Disease, will tend to experience impaired drug absorption and/or increased elimination of the drug from the GI tract.

The health and function of the liver and kidneys are extremely important for the normal removal of drugs and other toxic substances from the body. When drugs and their metabolites are not properly eliminated they tend to accumulate in the various organs and tissues of the body and produce adverse effects. Clients who present with either past or present disorders of these organs may be especially sensitive to the effects of drugs.

The health of the client can affect the amount of free drug in the blood. For example, clients who are fasting (unsupervised) or those with liver or kidney disease will often have a decrease in plasma albumin levels. Under these conditions, there will be more free drug to interact with target cells. If the dose of the drug is not modified the client is at risk for drug toxicity.

1. *1993 Compendium of Pharmaceutical Specialties*, 28th ed., Canadian Pharmaceutical Press, Ontario, Canada.

CHAPTER 5

General Treatment Guidelines

In Chapter 1 reference was made to a research study that investigated the combining of allopathic and complementary therapies by the American public. An important finding was that a large percentage of individuals did not inform their doctors that they were receiving complementary therapies while still under medical care.

Regardless of place of work or treatment style, today's massage therapists encounter many clients who are taking drugs. The potential for adverse interactions between a client's medications and the massage therapist's choice of treatment modalities, which could include hydrotherapy, stretching, deep tissue work, lymph drainage, and so on, must raise the question of client safety in the practitioner's mind. In treatment planning, the therapist must consider all factors that could compromise client safety; one such factor is medications.

Chapters 1 through 4 introduced the reader to basic concepts in pharmacology, including interpretation of key pharmacological terms, description of the routes of administration of medications, and discussion of some of the drug processing mechanisms in the body. When possible, an appropriate connection to massage therapy was made; for example, concerns were raised about the reliability of client feedback when an analgesic is being taken, and about the importance of understanding a drug's bioavailability and plasma levels in relation to scheduling treatments. To promote client safety, therapists need to have a basic understanding of pharmacologic principles, and the ability to interrelate this knowledge with the physiological effects of massage therapy modalities and approaches.

Let's look at a drug profile and relate the information to massage treatment planning. The following excerpt[1] contains information about the anticonvulsant (used in the treatment of epilepsy) drug carbamazepine.

"The absorption of carbamazepine in man is relatively slow. When taken in a single oral dose the carbamazepine tablets and chewable tablets yield peak plasma concentrations of unchanged carbamazepine within 4-24 hours. Only 2-3% of the dose, whether given singly or repeatedly, is excreted in the urine in unchanged form. The primary metabolite is the pharmacologically active 10, 11-epoxide. After repeated doses the elimination half-life of unchanged carbamazepine is 16-24 hours depending on the duration of the medication.

"Because the onset of potentially serious blood dyscrasias [abnormal conditions of blood cells] may be rapid, patients should be made aware of early toxic signs and symptoms of a potential hematological problem, as well as symptoms of dermatological or hepatic reactions.

If reactions such as fever, sore throat, rash, ulcers in the mouth, easy bruising, petechial or purpuric hemorrhage [purplish red spots caused by the release into the skin of a very small quantity of blood from a capillary] appear, the patient should be advised to contact his or her physician immediately.

"Other adverse reactions include: skin sensitivity reactions and rashes, photosensitivity, hypertension or hypotension, nausea, vomiting, and aggressive behavior."

How would a massage therapist use the above information and relate it to massage treatment?

- Since carbamazepine is used in the treatment of epilepsy, the stability of the client's condition is of concern. Treatments should be scheduled when peak levels of the drug are expected – according to the drug profile this occurs at least 4 hours after taking a dose.

- Good clinical practice would include taking a BP reading at the start of each treatment. If you observe significant changes, inform the client and suggest a follow up visit to the medical practitioner.

- The health and function of the liver and kidneys are extremely important for maintenance of therapeutic levels of medications in the blood. The long half-life of this drug, and the fact that the primary metabolite is pharmacologically active, suggest that the client can quickly develop adverse effects if normal elimination processes are compromised by poor organ health. Complaints such as fever, and reddish or purplish bruises as mentioned in the drug profile, are early indications of drug toxicity. The practitioner will want to stay alert to the symptoms and complaints of the client. When there are indicators of drug toxicity present, massage treatments are contraindicated until the client is evaluated and 'cleared' by the attending physician.

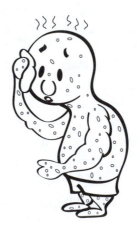

This chapter draws on information presented in earlier chapters and focuses on decision-making for the massage therapist, integrating clinical implications of clients' medication use into general guidelines for massage therapy that promote safe and effective treatment. These include guidelines for:

- assessment
- treatment planning
- hydrotherapy
- therapeutic exercise prescription and client self care
- treating around injection sites, skin patches, and implant devices

1.   GUIDELINES FOR ASSESSMENT

Most clients have a limited ability to distinguish the multitude of factors that can contribute to their symptoms. This is especially likely if the complaints are related to medication effects. If the massage therapist is unaware of the mechanisms of action of medications and the potential impact of side effects, interpretation of the client's symptom picture and assessment findings can lead to misleading conclusions. This in turn can result in development and administration of ineffective or harmful treatment plans and poor client recovery.

At the end of this section you will find a sample letter to a medical practitioner addressing a situation where the massage therapist believes a medication side effect may be contributing to a client's clinical presentation.

A client's medications have the potential to alter the results of the massage therapist's assessment of his or her case. In this section we will explore how drugs can affect:

- the client's complaints
- case history taking
- observation
- palpation
- movement examination/special and neurological testing

You will also be introduced to the Medication Case History Intake Form.

The Client's Complaints

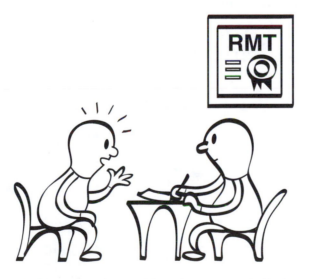

Listening to the client characterize the problem is an especially important part of conducting an assessment. With experience, the practitioner can often form an accurate clinical impression just by listening to the client's description of his or her complaint. When medication effects are contributing to a client's presentation, the therapist may notice that the symptoms and test results do not 'add up' to a typical diagnostic picture, or may be puzzled that the symptoms exceed or differ from what might be expected. These situations should be referred to the doctor for evaluation.

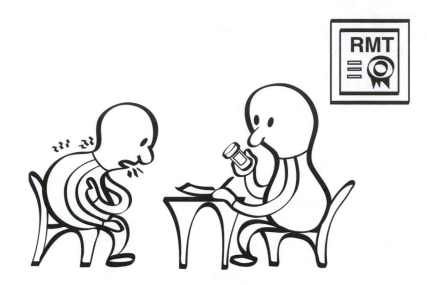

It is also true that medication side effects can mimic common complaints seen in massage therapy practice, for example headaches, fatigue, swollen ankles, and muscle and joint pain. This awareness can help the practitioner to anticipate the involvement of medications in some cases, or to follow through appropriately if massage treatment does not have the expected result in addressing the complaint.

The chart below gives examples of this type of overlap.

Side Effects That Mimic Common Complaints

Complaint	NSAIDs	Anti-Hypertensives	Corticosteroids	Anti-Depressants	Anti-Anxiety Meds
Headaches	yes	yes	yes	yes	yes
Drowsiness	yes	yes		yes	yes
Dizziness	yes	yes	yes	yes	yes
Fatigue	yes	yes	yes	yes	yes
Swollen ankles	yes	yes	yes		
Rash	yes	yes	yes	yes	yes
Numbness or tingling	yes	yes			
Muscle or joint pain		yes	yes	yes	

Case History Taking

In addition to having clients fill out general case history forms, it can be very useful to incorporate a specific form to document each client's medications, remedies, and supplements. Unless asked specifically, clients will often forget to inform you about some of the substances they are using. Those who are taking several types of over-the-counter (OTC) and/or prescribed medications may need to take the form home and check their medicine cabinets in order to complete the information as requested.

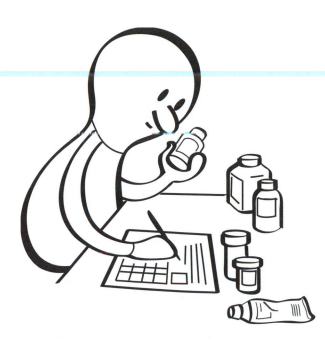

The reasons for having a medication case history form include:

- to have a clear record of which drugs and other substances are being taken and why

- to identify and initiate follow-up if the client does not know the reason for taking a drug

- to have a reference for sorting client complaints in light of potential relationships to medication use

- to identify if the drugs being used are from the same group (the client is potentially "double-dosing" and may be more predisposed to adverse reactions)

- to identify the full profile of what is being taken and the potential for multi-substance side effects (it can sometimes be enlightening to see how many drugs are being used by one person and to determine whether any one doctor is aware of the full profile)

- to have a quick reference for treatment planning

- as a service to the client – building a medication/remedy profile may prove helpful as a reference in the long-term management of his or her health

Medication Case History Intake Form*

On these two pages you will find a sample case history form specifically for medications, remedies, and supplements.

Medication Case History - Intake Form   Date _____

Your health and well-being are important to us, so please take a few moments to complete the form provided. The information will help us plan a safer and more effective treatment for you. **All information obtained will be confidential.**

NAME _____ AGE _____ OCCUPATION _____

ADDRESS _____

PHONE NUMBERS   (H) _____ (W) _____

FAMILY DOCTOR _____ PHONE _____

Within the last 4 weeks: YES   NO

Has your medical doctor prescribed any new medications or changed your medications?   ○   ○

Has your naturopath or medical herbalist prescribed any remedies for you?   ○   ○

Has your dentist prescribed any medications for you?   ○   ○

Have you purchased any over-the-counter items for health purposes from a pharmacy or health food shop?   ○   ○

Are you presently taking any herbal, Chinese medicine, or homeopathic remedies?   ○   ○

Are you presently taking any vitamin or mineral supplements?   ○   ○

	Name & Strength	Date Started	# Per Day	Reason for Use
List any prescribed or over-the-counter items you are presently taking orally:				
List any herbal, Chinese medicine, or homeopathic remedies you are presently taking orally:				
List any vitamin or mineral supplements you are presently taking orally:				

© 2001 Curties-Overzet Publications   To order: 1-888-649-5411   **p.t.o.**

	YES	NO	If yes, please answer the following:

Are you presently using any medicinal creams or ointments? ○ ○
Name of preparation: (1) _____ (2) _____
Reason for use: _____
Date started: _____
Area (on the body) of use: _____
How often do you apply it: _____

Are you presently using any medicinal eye, ear or nose preparations? ○ ○
Name of preparation: (1) _____ (2) _____
Reason for use: _____
Date started: _____
Area (on the body) of use: _____
How often do you apply it: _____

Are you presently using any skin patch preparation? ○ ○
Name of preparation: (1) _____ (2) _____
Reason for use: _____
Date started: _____
Area (on the body) of use: _____
How often do you apply it: _____

Are you presently using any medicinal preparation in the vagina or the rectum? ○ ○
Name of preparation: (1) _____ (2) _____
Reason for use: _____
Date started: _____
How often do you apply it: _____

Are you self-injecting any medication? (insulin, pain killers, testosterone, etc.) ○ ○
Name of preparation: (1) _____ (2) _____
Reason for use: _____
Date started: _____
Area (on the body) of injection: _____
How often do you self-inject: _____

Do you have any medication delivery implant devices? ○ ○
Name of preparation: (1) _____ (2) _____
Reason for use: _____
Date started: _____
Area and route of implantation: _____

Do you drink coffee or tea on a regular basis? ○ ○
If yes, how many cups per day: _____ or per week: _____

Do you drink alcoholic beverages on a regular basis? ○ ○
If yes, how many drinks per day: _____ or per week: _____

Do you smoke? ○ ○
If yes, how many packs per day: _____ or per week: _____

Within the last week have you used any recreational drugs? ○ ○

Have you experienced any of the following since starting the medication/natural remedy therapy?

☐ anxiety	☐ insomnia	☐ irritability	☐ blurred vision	☐ liver infection	☐ decreased appetite
☐ headaches	☐ joint pain	☐ drowsiness	☐ muscle aches	☐ yeast infection	☐ difficulty breathing
☐ fatigue	☐ depression	☐ swelling	☐ frequent flu	☐ difficult urination	☐ cold hands and feet
☐ dizziness	☐ confusion	☐ dry skin	☐ stomach pain	☐ high blood pressure	☐ shortness of breath
☐ fever	☐ nausea	☐ bitter taste	☐ athletes foot	☐ heart palpitations	☐ low blood pressure
☐ chills	☐ tremors	☐ loss of taste	☐ weight gain/loss	☐ increased tiredness	☐ prolonged menses
☐ bruising	☐ numbness	☐ skin rash	☐ muscle weakness	☐ bladder infection	☐ stomach irritation
☐ diarrhea	☐ vomiting	☐ constipation	☐ joint swelling	☐ kidney infection	☐ decreased sex drive
☐ hair loss	☐ tingling	☐ chest pain	☐ other: _____		

Are you allergic to any substances? (e.g. oils, drugs, aromas, metals, etc.) Yes ○ No ○ If yes, please specify:
_____

Additional Comments: _____

Signature: _____ Date: _____

* You may want to use this form as a reference in designing your own, or you can contact Curties-Overzet Publications to purchase these forms in bulk.

To enhance the usefulness of the information gathered on the medication intake form, therapists need to consider the impact of the following:

When more than one medication is prescribed for the treatment of a single condition, for example:

- Hypertension is often managed with a combination of diuretics and betablocker medications.

- Following soft tissue injury, muscle relaxants and anti-inflammatories are often prescribed together.

- The common flu is often managed with cough and cold medications, and sometimes antibiotics to treat/prevent secondary infections.

The combination of medications may cause an increased incidence of side effects or perhaps unpredictable effects experienced by the client.

A single medication can be used in the management of more than one condition, for example:

- Aspirin is normally recommended for mild to moderate pain; however, it is also increasingly used in the management of cardiovascular diseases for its anticoagulant effect.

- Corticosteroids are used in treating several conditions, including asthma, bronchitis, arthritis, ulcerative colitis, and various types of autoimmune and allergic disorders.

Therapists are encouraged to make sure it is clear why a particular medication is being used, and to assess whether there is more than one purpose for the client taking the drug. Knowing what the client is being treated for makes for better treatment planning.

When one or more of the medications is a long-term prescription:

- Long-term use of medications is an indication that the client's condition may be serious. Before treating, it is important to be clear about the nature and progression of the condition.

- Concerns arise about the health of the liver and kidneys, since these organs are responsible for the metabolism and elimination of drugs and are more likely to be compromised by long-term medication use. The client's symptoms/complaints may be related to accumulation of metabolites in the body. Inquire in detail about side effects that have been experienced, or might be anticipated.

- Long-term use of some medications can lead to the development of another pathology. For example, prolonged corticosteroid use can promote osteoporosis. Postmenopausal women and the elderly are especially predisposed.

- The health of the other body systems, i.e. the cardiovascular, respiratory, digestive, and so on, needs to be monitored ongoingly for stresses or side effects imposed by long-term medication use. As an example, long-term use of morphine for analgesia can cause constipation and long-term aspirin use can lead to ulcers.

- Several medications when taken long-term can reduce the integrity of the body's tissues, a particular concern for massage therapists. Be alert for dry/cracked skin, open lesions, edema, tissue dystrophy, and sensory impairment; assess for reduced resilience of connective tissue structures like ligaments and tendons. Ask for medical guidance as needed.

When the client is taking a mix of traditional and non-traditional substances:

Since there are many gaps in this area of knowledge, it is often not easy to find out about the potential interactions among medications and the remedies and supplements that many clients are taking. If the client is seeing another health care professional, for example a naturopath or homeopath, this person can be an important source of information. Existing studies can also be searched out at the library or on the Internet. A helpful website is www.onemedicine.com. An alert practitioner will always keep in mind the possibility that the client's clinical picture and assessment findings may be affected by such substance mixing.

Observation

Observation, or the 'looking phase,' begins when the therapist greets the client; it is an important source of information about the client's health. This part of an assessment includes observing for:

- facial expression
- gait and movement patterns
- skin color and health
- edema

- physical deformity
- standing and sitting posture
- limb size and shape

Let's look at an example of how a client's medication can affect the interpretation of observed information.

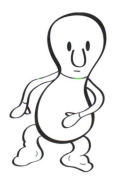

A client on long-term use of a calcium channel blocker medication will be predisposed to developing an altered gait pattern. This is because accumulation of edema in the feet and ankles is often associated with this group of drugs. The massage therapist who is unaware of this side effect may interpret the altered gait as caused by a hip or lower back disorder and plan a treatment to focus on these areas. The edema may be perceived as secondary rather than primary in the etiology of the problem.

To resolve the altered gait, and any secondary complaints of the client such as hip and lower back pain, the edema in the feet and ankles must be treated. As well, the physician needs to be informed of the degree to which the medication is affecting the client's musculoskeletal system.

Palpation

Changes in tissue health, muscle tone (hypo- or hypertonicity), skin temperature and moisture, fascial mobility, myofascial trigger points, and tissue fluid levels are all palpable by massage therapists.

Here are a few examples of how the use of medications can cause palpable changes:

- Muscle relaxants and other CNS depressants will alter the tone of the skeletal muscles so that they feel 'loose' and are too easily overstretched.

- Long-term use of oral corticosteroids will lead to breakdown of connective tissues including the skin, muscle, and lymphatic tissues. Edema may be present, the skin will often feel fragile, and muscles tend to be soft and hypotonic.

- Ibuprofen, an easily available anti-inflammatory, can cause increased perspiration. On palpation, the skin will feel cool and moist.

- Repeatedly used injection sites can feel edematous, nodular, and fibrotic, with fascial mobility restrictions; such sites can also be a source of pain.

Movement Examination/Special and Neurological Tests

During the testing portion of the assessment, the client is asked to perform certain movements and/or the therapist moves the client's body through special tests that target the structures being assessed. The test findings help determine which tissue structures are involved, and to what degree, in the presenting complaint.

Let's look at two examples of how medications can alter responses to movement and special tests:

- Medications such as anti-inflammatories and narcotic analgesics alter the client's pain perception. When asked to do active movements, the client may be able to perform normal or near normal range of motion without showing signs of pain and discomfort that would accurately reflect the stresses being applied to the tissues. Passive movement results are likely to be skewed in a similar fashion.

- Centrally acting skeletal muscle relaxants depress the CNS. The results of neurological testing on, for example, deep tendon reflexes, dermatomes, and myotomes will be altered. Responses of muscles to manual testing will be weakened and they will show signs of fatigue more easily.

Sample Letter to Medical Practitioner

The letter that follows is an example of the type of correspondence a massage therapist might send to the doctor of a shared client in a case where, from the therapist's viewpoint, a medication side effect may be playing a role in the client's presentation. It is important to keep in mind that such letters must be as brief as possible, well organized, and written in a neutral, professional tone.

Massage Therapy Center,
Suite 123, Femur Drive, Patellaville
Tel/Fax: 000-123-4567

November 12, 2001

Dr. Rectus Femoris
345 Adductor Drive,
Patellaville

RE: Possible Medication Side Effect

Dear Dr. Femoris,

I am writing in connection with a patient in your practice, Mr. Iliac Crest, who has recently begun receiving massage therapy.

Client's Complaint: Mr. Crest presented at my clinic two weeks ago complaining of right hip pain and sore, swollen ankles and feet. He described the hip pain as "dull and achy," occurring especially after activities involving prolonged standing or walking, and stated that the peripheral edema is most uncomfortable in the evenings.

Client History: Mr. Crest had his quarterly medical evaluation with you three months ago. As his blood pressure was up, you prescribed an additional antihypertensive medication, a calcium channel blocker. Six weeks ago Mr. Crest visited your clinic complaining of an achy right hip and tired feet. You prescribed an anti-inflammatory, ordered X-rays of the hip and lumbar spine, and suggested that he elevate his feet at the end of the day.

Clinical Assessment: Changes in gait and pelvic mobility patterns were observed. Bilateral leg edema was evident, with right side prominence. Orthopedic assessment revealed hypertonicity of the hip and lumbar musculature, but suggested no specific lesion. The anti-inflammatory did not reduce the symptoms. There is no history of trauma to the hip joint, and I understand the X-ray report indicated no abnormalities. Mr. Crest informed me that the swelling began about 4 weeks after his quarterly visit to you.

Clinical Impression: Mr. Crest's altered gait may be causing his hip pain and discomfort. As you know, peripheral edema can be a side effect of calcium channel blockers. The time frame links his symptom onset with beginning the new medication, as does the progression, with early symptoms of peripheral edema causing foot and ankle discomfort followed later by hip pain. The massage therapy sessions have been aimed at reducing the edema and addressing the increased muscle tone. Although temporary alleviation was effected, there has not been substantial improvement. I would be happy to provide additional information regarding the massage therapy sessions if you wish.

I look forward to hearing your decision in this matter.

Yours truly,

Tib Anterior, R.M.T.

2. GUIDELINES FOR TREATMENT PLANNING

Treatment planning involves being familiar with the general health of the client, having a good understanding of the nature and progression of the presenting condition(s), and designing a safe and effective approach to achieving the massage treatment goals.

The massage treatment plan should complement other types of care the client might be receiving. Providing safe and effective treatment compatible with a client's medications can be challenging for the practitioner. This section will elaborate several guidelines related to how drugs can affect:

- the scheduling of treatments
- treatment focus and duration
- techniques used during treatment
- client cooperativeness

Drugs Can Affect Treatment Scheduling

It is beyond the massage therapist's scope of practice to tell clients when to take their medications. However, by adjusting when massage therapy is given, the practitioner can work to best coincide treatment with the bioavailablity cycles of drug use.

Let's look at two important considerations:

• Medical Stability of the Client

A client whose condition necessitates long-term drug use usually requires a certain medication level in the blood to ensure that the condition remains stable. Here are a few examples:

- an insulin dependent diabetic must have regular doses of insulin to maintain acceptable levels of glucose in the blood
- a client being treated for a chronic pain syndrome requires pain medication for physical and emotional stability
- an epileptic client needs to maintain peak blood levels of anticonvulsant medication to stabilize the central nervous system and reduce the likelihood of seizures

Treatment planning must take into account that the circulatory and neural effects of massage therapy may tend toward destabilizing this type of client. In addition to judicious treatment modification, the practitioner should consider scheduling treatment sessions at a medication-appropriate time **after** the client's scheduled dosage. The purpose is to ensure maximal bioavailability of the medication, and therefore better stability of the client during and after the treatment.

- **Client Feedback Implications**

As previously discussed, drugs such as non-steroidal anti-inflammatories, narcotic analgesics, and central nervous system depressants can alter a client's ability to give accurate feedback about the comfort of techniques and modalities used during massage treatment. These medications alter normal pain responses that warn of potential tissue injury. Techniques or modalities that would normally cause some discomfort become more tolerable than they should.

Consider a client taking an anti-inflammatory for a few days because of a minor injury. The client seeks massage therapy to assist with the healing process; however, the drug's analgesic properties will compromise the client's ability to comment on what the injured tissues are experiencing during the treatment. The client, who has a reduced perception of pain, provides misleading information to the therapist, saying things like "you can go deeper if you want." If the therapist responds by doing deeper massage in such a situation, there is a likelihood of causing more tissue damage and promoting more bruising.

For clients taking medications short-term for minor conditions, recommended treatment scheduling is **just before or soon after** the medication dose. With lower bloodstream bioavailability of the drug the client is likely to give more accurate feedback about the techniques and modalities used. However, the massage therapist should still be cautious since the drug's onset of action can mask symptoms of overtreatment. If unsure about how to judge the ideal timing of a massage treatment for tissue safety, the therapist is encouraged to discuss this concern with the client and/or the attending physician.

Drugs Can Require Adapting/Shortening the Treatment

- **Energy Level of the Client**

Fatigue is a common side effect of many medications, including the hypertension medications, anti-anxiety drugs, and many of the antidepressants. In this case massage therapy may cause even more fatigue, and a shorter, more specific treatment design is needed. The client should be asked to monitor during and after treatments for decreased energy or other adverse effects, so that the massage therapist can evolve a treatment design most suited to the circumstance.

- **Emotional Stability of the Client**

Long-term use of some drugs, for example corticosteroids, is associated with mood fluctuations; depression and anxiety are side effects of many medications. It is possible that with the additional physical/emotional effects of massage therapy, some clients may feel emotionally volatile or overwhelmed, and this may warrant ending the treatment early or planning for shorter sessions. Discuss this possibility with the client in advance and together develop a plan of action.

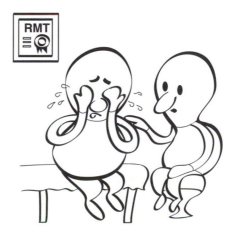

Drugs Can Influence the Selection of Manual Techniques

Many medications will influence how manual techniques are to be applied during a massage session. In the chapters that follow, as drug group applications are discussed in more detail, more specific guidelines will be elaborated on. Let's look here at some examples that give rise to general guidelines:

• Some Drugs Alter Blood Clotting Mechanisms

Clients will be predisposed to bruising when taking medications that alter the normal blood clotting process. Examples include anticoagulants, platelet inhibitors, and aspirin and the other non-steroidal anti-inflammatory drugs.

Massage techniques like muscle stripping, deep kneading, ischemic compressions (for trigger point therapy), and cross fiber frictions must be modified or avoided. These techniques, when used on normal healthy connective tissue to promote good fiber alignment, often produce a mild inflammatory response that is easily resolved. However, when the client is taking a medication with anticoagulant properties they can result in excessive bruising and inflammation.

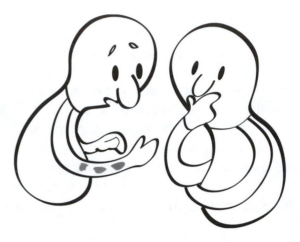

• Some Drugs Alter Protective Responses

Several medications, including centrally acting muscle relaxants, narcotic analgesics, and anti-anxiety drugs, depress nervous system reactions to sensory feedback from the stretch and tension receptors in muscle and joint tissues. Firing from these sensory organs (muscle spindle, golgi tendon organ, joint capsule and ligament receptors) may not elicit expected responses to techniques that place stress or stretch on them. Massage therapists tend to rely on such responses to determine when the pressure is deep enough or a stretch is being applied optimally. When the tissue does not tighten as a signal, manual techniques can inadvertently be applied too aggressively and tissue damage caused. Techniques such as aggressive contract-relax stretching and deep tissue work must be eliminated from the treatment plan, or used very cautiously.

While the usual effect is to reduce the potency of protective reflexes, in some cases overreactions can occur, leading to muscle spasm and reflex muscle guarding.

• Some Drugs Compromise Tissue Integrity

The corticosteroids in particular, especially when used long term, cause atrophy and weakening of skin, ligaments, joint capsules, bones, and muscles and their tendons. When injected into joints for arthritic conditions, they can induce breakdown of articular cartilage.

Any massage approaches that involve placing direct pressure or stress on tissue structures will need to be employed carefully. Techniques such as rib springing, heavy tapotement, passive forced stretching, muscle stripping, deep kneading, frictions, and joint mobilization should be significantly modified or avoided. Be particularly careful with clients who are at risk for developing osteoporosis, for example post-menopausal women and the elderly.

Normal health, function, and sensitivity of the skin are also compromised by prolonged topical corticosteroid use. Skin rolling, frictions, and wringing techniques can result in bruising and inflammation of the subcutaneous tissues.

The therapist should note that the conditions caused by such medication use will also impair repair processes in body tissues, resulting in healing time frames that are often longer than the 'norm' and prolonged tissue fragility after injury.

- **Some Drugs Mask Pain Responses**

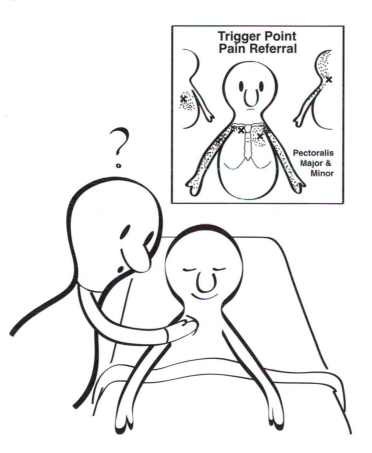

Since assessment results can be compromised in the absence of normal pain sensation, the test findings of clients using anti-inflammatories or analgesics, either orally or topically, can make their tissues appear more healthy and resilient than they truly are. The unaware practitioner may plan to use more aggressive treatment techniques than is appropriate. It is important to rely less on client feedback and more on observation and palpation, as well as on medical advice as needed.

Drugs Can Alter a Client's Cooperativeness

Various drugs, especially those that depress the central nervous system like the narcotic analgesics and anti-anxiety agents, can make a client less communicative and seemingly indifferent to supplying information in a complete way, either during case history taking or in the course of treatment. The therapist will often need to spend more time and take a determined approach, asking specific questions and making sure that feedback is frequently solicited.

3. GUIDELINES FOR HYDROTHERAPY

Hydrotherapy is generally defined as "the use of water in any of its three forms, solid, liquid and gas, used internally or externally for a therapeutic response." All physiologic systems of the body are influenced in one way or another by the combination of hydrotherapy modalities and medications. Since hydrotherapy is a common component of massage therapy treatment plans, and practitioners often suggest hydrotherapy as home care, an appreciation of how client medication use impacts on hydrotherapy decisions is important.

This section will look at how the concurrent use of drugs can affect:

- blood vessel reactions to hot and cold stimuli

- sensitivity of the skin to temperature changes

- the body's temperature control mechanisms

Some Drugs Alter How Blood Vessels React to Hot and Cold

Blood vessels generally react to hot applications by dilating (vasodilation), to brief cold applications by constricting (vasoconstriction), and to prolonged cold by first constricting and then dilating. Contrast applications (alternating hot and cold) cause the blood vessels to alternately vasodilate and vasoconstrict, and are aimed at strengthening vasomotor functions. Factors that influence the nature or degree of any of these reactions will alter responses to hydrotherapy modalities.

Let's consider the following scenario:

A client is diagnosed with moderate hypertension, work-related stress being a major contributing factor. On the recommendation of a friend the client visits a local day spa for some relaxation therapy. After review of the treatments offered, the decision is made to proceed with a 20-minute hot tub followed by a full body massage.

The client is taking an antihypertensive medication that lowers blood pressure by causing dilation of the peripheral blood vessels. During the hot tub the client begins to feel lightheaded, and on emerging from it complains to the massage therapist of dizziness, fatigue, nausea, and headache. These symptoms relate to the combined effects of the antihypertensive

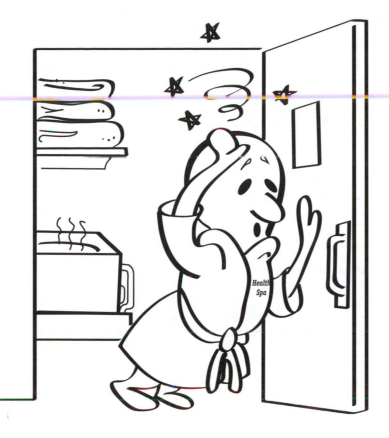

medication and the systemic heat application. Massage therapy might heighten these effects and is no longer indicated.

The hydrotherapy choice in this situation is not appropriate given the medication use, and if the spa therapists are unaware of such implications, client safety can be compromised. In addition to antihypertensive medications, several other drugs, including for example the narcotic analgesics, also cause peripheral vasodilation.

Some drugs act on receptors in blood vessel walls to cause vasoconstriction. They are used:

- to treat migraine headaches – e.g. sumatriptan (Imitrex)
- for congestion (ephedrine and pseudoephedrine are commonly found in decongestant preparations)
- to treat children with Attention Deficit Hyperactivity Disorder (ADHD) – methylphenidate (Ritalin)
- to promote weight loss, e.g. a CNS stimulant like dextroamphetamine (Dexedrine)
- in medical emergencies, for example shock, hypotension, and other types of circulatory emergencies, to increase blood pressure
- in topical anaesthetic preparations to extend the time period that the anaesthetizing agent stays in the area

When the vasodilation capacity of blood vessels is compromised by drug use, all extreme temperature hydrotherapy is contraindicated. With hot applications, the normal dilation response helps distribute the heat evenly through the tissue and tends to prevent burning at the site of application. Blood vessels that are held in constriction are less effective in this role and the client may be burned. On the other hand, if a cold modality is used, the constricted blood vessels may respond to the application by going into spasm. This leads to tissue ischemia and can be quite painful.

When drugs are influencing the contractility of blood vessel walls to impair either vasoconstriction or vasodilation responsiveness, hydrotherapy modalities must be moderated and cautiously applied.

Some Drugs Change Skin Sensitivity to Temperature

Skin receptors play an important role in the interpretation of hot and cold sensations. Prolonged topical corticosteroid use, local skin creams and ointments used for muscle and joint pain, and CNS depressant medications can cause decreased sensitivity of the skin to temperature stimuli.

Consider another client, who regularly complains of anxiety-related headaches and a stiff shoulder, and is taking prescribed anti-anxiety medication twice daily, codeine tablets for headache, and using a topical OTC analgesic rub for the shoulder discomfort.

This client presents for massage treatment complaining of the sore shoulder and of interscapular pain. On palpation, the shoulder and periscapular muscles feel hypertonic, and there is decreased mobility of the local vertebral and costovertebral joints. The therapist applies a hot pack for 15 minutes before beginning manual treatment. The combined effects of the oral and topical medications have the potential to reduce the client's ability to 'feel' the hot pack. Tissue sensation will become even more inexact, risking burning, and feedback about the manual techniques used next will be additionally compromised. Since the therapist will not receive accurate feedback about the hydrotherapy application or the subsequent massage work, the client will probably be bruised and in more pain the next day.

Some Drugs Alter the Body's Temperature Control Mechanisms

Medications like the phenothiazines (used in psychiatric medicine) suppress the hypothalamic centers that regulate central and peripheral temperature control mechanisms. Homeostatic regulation of body temperatures is affected.

In both hot/humid and hot/dry conditions the ability of the body to sweat and thereby cool itself can be reduced. Hydrotherapy modalities like steams, saunas, hot baths, and sweating herbal wraps produce similar conditions. Clients are at risk for developing heat intolerance, indicated by symptoms such as confusion, inability to sweat, hot dry skin, nausea, and muscle weakness.

The chilled client can pose a similar concern. For example, therapists working at ski resorts see clients who have spent the day on the slopes and are complaining of feeling chilled. It makes sense to warm them up with a steam or hot tub. If any of these clients are taking medications that alter body temperature controls, the choice of warming hydrotherapy must be much more moderate, incorporating modified application temperature and a less full body focus.

In addition to steams and hot tubs, cold plunges are becoming more popular at spas and other destination resorts. Cold plunge modalities are contraindicated for any client taking medications that alter body temperature control mechanisms.

Quick Guide to Hydrotherapy Case History Questions

In addition to asking directly about a client's medication related hydrotherapy effects, general information elicited in case history taking may point to hydrotherapy concerns that need more follow up. This can be significant in helping amalgamate all the case information to create a safe and effective treatment plan.

- the client's preferences related to hot and cold – are there any medically advised hydrotherapy or temperature restrictions?

- blood pressure and pulse – what is normal for the client? is the BP high or low? requiring medication control?

- daily bath or shower temperatures (use as a guide for what is being well tolerated when making hydrotherapy application decisions)

- areas of impaired circulation, including cold hands/feet, varicosities

- areas of sensory deficit

- time of last meal, for two reasons;

  - if the last meal was more than 6 hours ago full body modalities such as herbal baths or steam treatments will increase the cellular metabolic rate and can cause a drop in blood sugar levels

  - full body hydro treatments should be delayed at least 2 hours after a large meal

- past experience with hydrotherapy – reactions to previous treatments?

- the condition of the skin and underlying connective tissues

- allergies or sensitivities to essential oils, bath additives, etc.

- pregnancy: what trimester, any medical restrictions related to temperature use, blood pressure problems?

- presence of systemic conditions such as fibromyalgia, lupus, diabetes, cancer, respiratory conditions (asthma, emphysema, bronchitis), circulatory or cardiovascular problems including angina, stroke, etc.

Quick Guide to Hydrotherapy Treatment Modifications

This information is offered to assist the therapist in making hydrotherapy choices and monitoring client reactions to treatment in order to minimize adverse occurrences.

Options for modifying hydrotherapy treatments to reduce their intensity include:

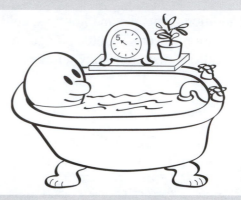

- <u>shorter duration:</u> Each treatment has a customary duration. For example, herbal baths generally last 10-20 minutes. Clients recovering from conditions like the flu can benefit from the effects of an herbal bath, but may still be on antibiotics or other medications and will be generally weakened. Shorter treatment times are recommended.

- <u>local hydrotherapy versus systemic:</u> A client who is recovering from a sinus infection can benefit from the effects of steam on the respiratory system. During the recovery period a local treatment like a facial steam may be less fatiguing than a systemic treatment like a medicated steam bath.

- <u>modified treatment temperatures:</u> Although each treatment modality has its 'ideal' temperature, modifying the temperature/temperature range can make hydrotherapy applications more enjoyable and safer for the client. For example:

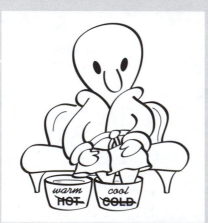

1. With contrast hydrotherapy treatments, the greater the temperature difference between the hot and cold applications, the more intense the effects on the blood vessels. Strong contrast hydrotherapy applications involve temperature differentials of 10-40 C (50-104 F). A factor like long-term use of corticosteroid medication can affect the health and contractile ability of the blood vessels, and suggests temperature modifications to somewhere in the 20-30 C range (68-86 F) would be more appropriate.

2. A systemic treatment like a medicinal/herbal bath is usually administered at 36-38 C, 97-100 F. At this temperature there will be an elevation of the body's basal metabolic rate, which potentially increases the workload of the heart. For the hypertensive client or client with a weakened heart, this can be cause for concern. Such clients will benefit from a tepid or neutral bath (35-36 C, 95-97 F).

Recognizing and Handling an Adverse Reaction to a Hydrotherapy Treatment

If a client reports feeling lightheaded/dizzy, experiencing nausea, or getting a headache, or if the skin becomes swollen, blotchy, or marbled (red/blue spots), stop the application immediately. Place the client in a comfortable rest position in a neutral temperature environment and provide room temperature water to be drunk in sips. Stay close and monitor for signs of improvement. Milder adverse reactions, especially when recognized early, usually begin to reverse in a short period of time; more serious reactions, or unusually prolonged ones, should be evaluated medically.

4. GUIDELINES FOR THERAPEUTIC EXERCISE PRESCRIPTION AND CLIENT SELF CARE

The overall goal of any exercise or self care program is to return the client to normal pain-free activities of daily living (ADLs). Exercises suggested by the massage therapist should complement any other medically supervised program. Self care activities for clients with systemic conditions such as hypertension, asthma, multiple sclerosis, or those recovering from a stroke or heart attack, should be developed closely with the medical team, physiotherapist, or qualified exercise trainer.

Exercise intolerance or adverse reactions to exercise include breathing difficulty, palpitations, chest pain, dizziness, nausea, vomiting, lightheadedness, or other symptoms that cause alarm.

There are a few simple generic guidelines to consider when suggesting an exercise program:

- give one or two activities at a time and monitor how the client responds
- develop a progressive exercise plan; begin with mild activities and progress to more challenging types
- develop the exercise plan around the client's lifestyle

The client's medication use can impact on exercise prescription by influencing the:

- desired frequency, intensity, and duration of the exercises
- time of day the exercises should be performed
- medical stability of client while performing the exercises

Some Drugs Will Influence Exercise Frequency, Intensity, and Duration (FID)

When introducing an activity such as walking, your instructions to the client might be: "Take a moderately paced [intensity] walk around your neighborhood block. It should be no longer than 10-15 minutes [duration] once a day for a week [frequency]."

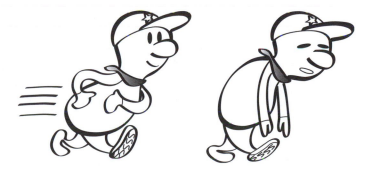

Exercise prescription needs to take into account the physiological effects that medications can have on the client's body. Fatigue, low energy, drowsiness, and muscle weakness are common drug side effects. As well, clients who are taking medications that depress the CNS or mask pain symptoms (for example, muscle relaxants and analgesics) will be at risk to injure or re-injure tissues if an aggressive exercise plan is recommended.

Some Drugs Influence the Time of Day Exercises Should Be Performed

Exercising in bright sunlight or on hot humid days can be quite risky when using certain medications. For example, clients taking medications in the phenothiazine family often experience sensitivity to sunlight. The metabolites from these medications accumulate in the skin and react with the sunlight to produce a deep blue-black discoloration. Clients who are predisposed to photosensitivity reactions should plan their activities for early morning or wait until later in the day, should exercise inside or in shaded areas, and should wear a hat and be well clothed when outdoors. Exercising in direct sunlight is not recommended.

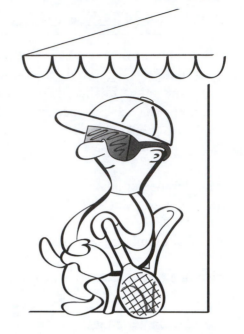

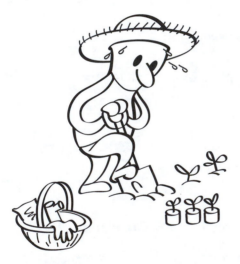

As previously mentioned, drugs like the phenothiazines also affect the temperature control mechanisms in the hypothalamus. Vigorous exercise on hot humid days is not recommended since there is increased risk of developing heat stroke.

Other drug groups that can cause photosensitivity reactions include antibiotics, sulfa drugs, muscle relaxants, and asthma medications. While it is difficult to predict who will experience these reactions, and how intensely, the elderly and very young are most at risk for adverse responses.

Some Drugs Impact the Medical Stability of the Exercising Client

Clients with systemic conditions like asthma, diabetes, and hypertension require special consideration in exercise program planning. For example, since exercise increases metabolic demands on the body, it is usually best for the insulin dependent diabetic client to exercise soon after taking his or her medication to ensure an adequate blood glucose level for cellular function.

Asthmatic clients need to keep triggering factors at a minimum when exercising. For example, it would not make sense to advocate swimming for a client who reacts to cold water or chlorine, or running through the woods at a high pollen time of year. Prescribed exercises should avoid exposures that tend to trigger asthma attacks as well as being well suited to the effects of the drugs the client is taking. The practitioner needs to ask about the client's medical guidelines for medication use and exercise and suggest compatible activities.

Some asthmatics cannot exercise at all without medication support. In these cases, it is best to rely on the exercise regime prescribed by the physician and/or physiotherapist.

Antihypertensive medications like the diuretics, vasodilators, and calcium channel blockers often produce side effects of joint pain, cramps, difficult breathing, fatigue, and reduced tolerance of heat. Clients who are using medications for heart disease and blood pressure control must be carefully monitored during any exercise program.

5. GUIDELINES FOR TREATING AROUND INJECTION SITES, SKIN APPLICATIONS, AND IMPLANT DEVICES

Treating on or around injection sites, skin patches, and implanted devices poses a challenge for massage therapists because not much is known about how massage and hydrotherapy modalities affect the release or uptake of medication from these sites. The information that is available can sometimes add to the sense of confusion. For example:

> "Massage of subcutaneous insulin injection sites markedly increased the absorption rate of insulin."[2]

> "Contrary to what might have being expected, our study of local massage suggests that the maneuver caused delay in the absorption of drug [fluphenazine decanoate] for at least the first hour."[3]

> A Japanese study[4] on massage during epidural block reports: "We conclude that peripheral sensory stimulation as weak as gentle massage may initiate a series of indirect mechanisms that lead to accelerated regression of sensory analgesia."

Taking the side of caution, it makes sense for massage therapists to assume that any manipulation on or around such a site, in particular an injection site or skin patch, has the potential to alter the pharmacokinetics of the drug being administered.

Injection sites can also be locations of tissue damage and degenerative change, posing concerns about how resilient the tissue is, how best to work with the tissue, and when to avoid local treatment:

> "If you received a cortisone type injection, make sure that you protect that area from hard exercise for at lease two months after you receive the injection."[5]

> "Certain drugs, especially the lipid (fat) soluble drugs, seem to cause direct damage to the muscle cell membrane resulting in muscle fiber necrosis."[6] (Although this study was done on laboratory animals, the implication for human tissue cannot be ignored.)

This section will explore the issues related to assessing and treating around injection sites, skin applications, and implant devices, including how to:

- assess the medication site

- recognize adverse reactions at the site

Guidelines will then be suggested for the practitioner to follow when working with clients who have cutaneous or subcutaneous medication sites.

Assessing the Medication Site

The practitioner must perform a thorough assessment before making decisions about whether/how to treat at or near a medication site. A good assessment will include:

- case history questions

- observation of the site

- palpation on and around the site

- movement assessment of the area

The therapist's questions are intended to elicit specific information about the reason for the injection, skin patch, or implant device, and any related concerns or medical guidelines. Close observation of the site will detect signs of inflammation, irritation, infection, bruising, or skin reactions; palpation and movement assessment give the therapist more detailed information about the health and strength of the connective tissues around the site.

Case History Questions

- reason for injection/patch/implanted device

- location of the site(s) – remember, some devices have entry and exit sites

- if a patch or implanted device, how long has it been there? is it changed or replaced regularly?

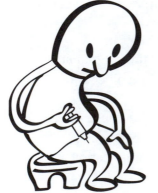

- if a regular injection site, how often is it used?

- are alternate sites used for injections? where? (e.g. diabetic client)

- when injections are administered, method of administration: intramuscular, intravenous, intra-articular, etc.

- is the injection self-administered, or administered by medical personnel?

- how long does the effect of the injection last?

- inquire about any side effects experienced currently or previously

- any history of infection at the site? if yes, what was the treatment and management? how long did it take to resolve?

- ask about any related abnormal sensation, muscle weakness, etc.

- any previous injections/patches/devices – reason for use, site of application, how long ago, etc.

Observation

- compare the body part/body area bilaterally

- is the site inflamed? does it look irritated?

- are there any signs of bruising, skin rashes, etc.

- does the skin look unusually dry or moist?

- is there any swelling proximal or distal to the site?

- is the site discolored?

- does the client show signs of apprehension or protectiveness of the site?

Palpation

Using thoroughly washed hands, or gloves:

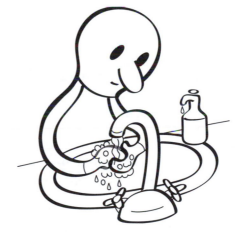

- compare the body part/body area bilaterally

- clearly identify the boundaries of the patch or device

- palpate around the site, not over the site – does palpation cause pain? (note your depth of palpation)

- assess for loss of sensation – can the client 'feel' you palpating?

- assess for edema; if present, gently push into the edema – is it pitted?

- does the skin feel unusually hot, dry, moist?

- does the tissue surrounding the site feel dense or fibrotic?

- what is the tissue mobility like – normal, loose, taut, fragile, adhered?

- palpate the local musculature – any pain or discomfort?

Movement Assessment

A movement assessment of the medication site typically involves the therapist assessing active (AROM), passive (PROM) and resisted (RROM) ranges of motion. If the test area seems irritated, instruct the client to move only within pain tolerance.

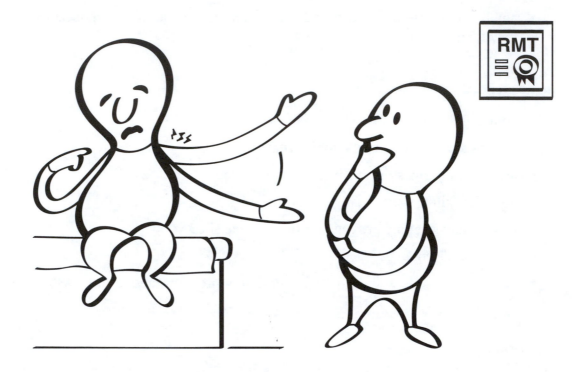

- AROM: The client performs active movements. For example, if the injection was given in the middle deltoid, having the client perform shoulder abduction helps the therapist assess the strength and degree of irritation of the deltoid muscle and its supporting connective tissue.

- PROM: The therapist moves the part and assesses for articular and connective tissue compliance, and range and smoothness of movement. Passive testing is especially indicated for intra-articular injections.

- RROM: The therapist resists the client's movements. If the site is not irritated, or is an old site, this will assess muscle integrity and strength and is especially indicated for intramuscular injections. RROM is not indicated if the site is inflamed or irritated.

The therapist needs to use common sense and professional judgment when performing movement testing; if apprehension or pain are elicited, discontinue and reassess at a later time. If the site has not been examined medically, in most instances the client should be advised to have it checked.

Adverse Reactions at the Medication Site

The most common adverse reactions at the medication site involve irritation, inflammation, or infection. Therapists can be alert to the following:

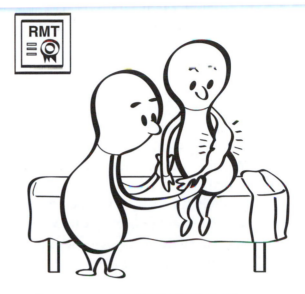

- If an injection is administered IM, the drug substance may be a source of irritation to the muscle tissue. This can lead to inflammation at the site. At sites located near nerves, for example, the gluteals and the sciatic nerve, nerve irritation may be the source of the symptoms (numbness, tingling, muscle weakness, radiating pain, etc.). Injections into rectus intermedius can lead to fibrosis and decreased knee flexion. Fibrosed injection sites may be tender and sensitive to touch.

- If an injection is administered IV, the drug substance may cause irritation of the vein wall, leading to thrombophlebitis. The site will be inflamed, with local and distal edema, and the client will experience discomfort.

- With injections administered intra-articularly, sometimes an almost immediate inflammatory reaction will occur. A possible reason for this is excessive immune reaction to the drug.

- Implanted devices can promote a variety of adverse reactions. Given that they consist of 'foreign' materials implanted through the skin into the tissues below, tissue irritation, infection, and hypersensitivity reactions can occur.

- Adverse reactions to skin patches are usually hypersensitivity responses.

Clinical Guidelines

The following guidelines are suggested for treating on or around injection sites, implanted devices, or other skin applications:

In General:

1. Carefully observe and palpate around the medication site for signs of inflammation, and to determine sensitivity. Be conscientious about hygiene. Assess the site at the start of each treatment.

   - If the site looks red and irritated, leave it alone.
   - If infection or inflammation has occurred, determine for how long and

what course of treatment has been pursued medically. The client may be on antibiotic or anti-inflammatory medications.

- Exercise caution if the client develops a fever, which can sometimes be caused by injections, for example flu shots. The presence of a fever indicates that the body is already working hard to mount an immune response and the additional stimulus of massage may be too taxing.

2.   If there is sensory impairment at a medication site, your approach to treatment will always be more cautious. Work on a small tissue area and monitor the response before planning deeper or more specific treatments.

3.   When working with a client in a hospital or private care setting, ensure that the attending physician or supervising nurse is aware of your visit. Follow the institutional guidelines for cleanliness, equipment checks, lubricant use, and so on. Do not remove any external applications from the client like IV lines, catheters, or electrodes. Also, keep in mind that your client may be immunocompromised, so if you feel a 'bug' coming on it is best to cancel your visit and reschedule when you are no longer contagious.

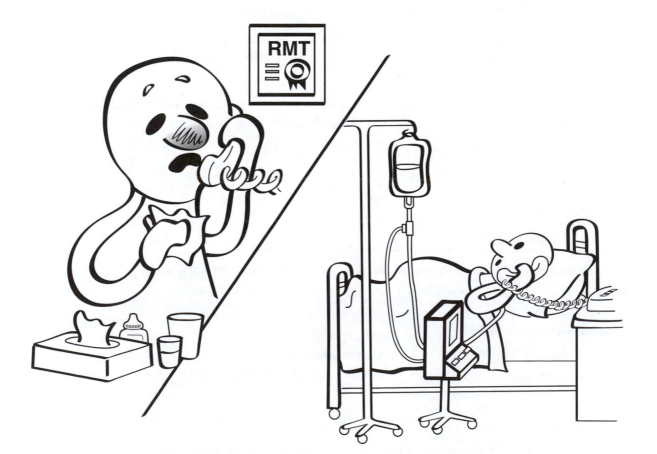

For Injection Sites:

1.   Thrombophlebitis can occur with IV injections. Working over or local to the site is contraindicated until the doctor indicates that the risk of embolism has subsided (thrombus detaches from the site and occludes a distant blood vessel, resulting in tissue death).

2.   When intramuscular injections are administered, the muscle tissue may be sore and inflamed for several days following the injection. Local massage should be avoided during this phase. Inquire about what instructions were given for managing the inflammation.

3.   When short acting injections are used, such as for vaccinations or local anaesthetic, the drug is typically absorbed and removed from the site within a few hours to a few days. If clear of all contraindications, an injection site can usually be included in the treatment after 24 to 48 hours. Safe techniques that can be used over the site include superficial fascial techniques, gentle stroking, vibrations, lymphatic drainage, and light petrissage.

4.   If the injection is long acting (a depot shot), do not perform any massage over the site. Consult with the physician about the type of drug used and how long it can be expected to stay within the tissues (can be as long as 6 weeks). Massaging over such sites while the drug is still being stored there is contraindicated.

5.   Infants who have immunization shots (intervals between 2 to 18 months) often develop a fever. If there is a fever, even a slight one, do not massage until it has resolved. If the site begins to show signs of irritation, follow the guidelines as discussed above.

6.   More focused work on the tissue at a site should wait a minimum of 10 days from discontinuation of use, or longer depending on the tissue recovery time frame in the case. If an older site is painful on palpation, refrain from treating it for a while longer to see if the pain subsides. If an older site is pain free, ensure that sensation in the tissue area is adequate and that the tissue at the site is in fact not more fragile than it appears.

7.   Older sites often feel adhered and fibrosed, especially if they were used repeatedly (e.g. diabetic client). As a general guideline, when working on an older fibrotic injection site begin cautiously with lighter work and then progress gradually to introduce hydrotherapy applications and more specific deeper techniques appropriate to achieving the goals of treatment. The client should be advised to monitor the site following each treatment for any adverse reactions such as inflammation, soreness, or bruising. Some reaction to focused work at the site would be expected, but if the post-treatment effects are stronger than you consider appropriate, reduce the intensity of the treatment approach.

8.   Use of hydrotherapy over injection sites: Application of heat over an injection site or implanted depot preparation will increase blood flow into the local tissues. This can

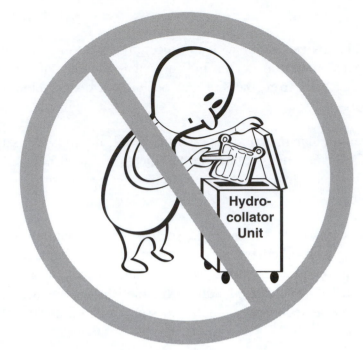

potentially speed uptake of the drug from the site, causing too much to be released into the bloodstream. The client will likely experience adverse effects as a result. For example, if a hot pack is placed over a recent insulin injection site, insulin will enter the blood too quickly and the likelihood is that the client will develop signs of hypoglycemia. Cold, on the other hand, produces local vasoconstriction and can cause reduced absorption of medication into the bloodstream, decreasing the rate of drug delivery to target sites. This can also lead to adverse effects. Although little research is available in this area, therapists must carefully consider the potential impact of hydrotherapy over injection sites and other topical and implant devices. Exercise professional judgment, and if unsure about the impact of a proposed hydrotherapy application, discuss your plan with the attending medical professional.

For Implanted Devices:

1.   When working with a client who has an implanted device, the therapist is responsible for exercising professional judgment at all times. It is important to ask as many questions as are needed to understand the type of drug being delivered and its effects, and the nature and operation of the device. Don't hesitate to check in with the attending physician if unsure about anything.

2.   Have the client clearly outline the implant's location and all of its attachment points. Working outside a 4-6 inch radius of the path of the device is suggested. When treating around these devices check in regularly with the client regarding comfort and tolerance of the treatment approach.

3.   The main concern is the risk of infection developing at the device's incision points. Excellent hygienic practices are absolutely necessary.

For Skin Patches:

1.   When a skin patch is present, a similar guideline of working outside a 4-6 inch radius of the patch is suggested. Performing massage techniques directly over the patch is contraindicated. It is unclear how massage will affect the pharmacokinetics of the imbedded drug, but the likelihood is that it could speed uptake of what is intended to be a time-released medication.

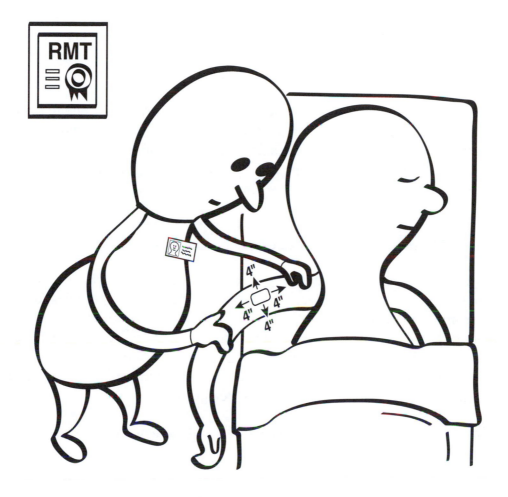

2.   The client should never be asked to remove the patch to give the practitioner access to work on the tissue below. Any such request is outside the massage therapy scope of practice. In addition, some patches are delivering medications (e.g., nitroglycerine for angina patients) that are necessary to the client's medical stability. Other types of applications (e.g., for birth control or quitting smoking) should also not be interrupted.

3.   The therapist needs to be aware that directly manipulating the patch can result in his or her skin surface being exposed to the drug, with the consequent risk of being 'dosed.' Since patches are often placed on the back of the arm and similar less visible areas, it is important to know and remember their locations to avoid inadvertently 'massaging' them.

Summary of General Massage Therapy & Medications Guidelines

1.   A thorough case history and assessment of the client is always necessary to obtain specific information about the client's use of medications, herbs, vitamins, and so on. This information is important for planning safe and appropriate treatments.

2.   Research the client's medications by reading the drug profiles. Take note of the mechanisms of action and potential side effects in each instance. Keep in mind that the more drugs and other substances a client is taking, the greater the likelihood of complex or idiosyncratic interactions. Consult with the doctor and other prescribing practitioners as needed to get a clearer picture.

3.   The therapist should always be alert to the possibility that a client's complaint or symptom presentation may be an effect or side effect of medication use. Reflect on the information you have gathered about the medications being taken, as well as medication start dates in relation to symptom onset. Consider whether there are indicators of drug toxicity.

4.   Remember that assessment results can be altered due to medication effects or side effects. Drugs that mask pain can create misleading test results.

5.   Be prepared to contact the attending physician or health care provider if you perceive a possible connection between medication effects and the client's complaints. Sometimes the assessment results will appear 'skewed,' or the client will not be benefiting from your treatment approach as expected. Create an open line of communication to discuss such concerns. When communicating with other practitioners, either verbally or in writing, be brief and well organized in presenting the information and maintain a balanced perspective.

6.   Consider whether the client's medication should influence your treatment scheduling. There are two key issues here:

   • maximizing bioavailability of drugs needed to stabilize the client's medical condition during and after the massage

   • maximizing the client's ability to give feedback during the treatment

7.   Consider carefully the physiologic effects of the client's medications from the perspective of how safely and effectively they would combine with the effects of your proposed treatment plan components.

8.   When using hydrotherapy modalities, monitor the tissue responses closely, along with the client's overall comfort level. When uncertain how well the application will be tolerated, begin cautiously and assess the response during and post treatment. It is better to use a well-tolerated modality that is gentler than is customary than to precipitate adverse effects.

9.	Ensure that any exercises you suggest are compatible with the client's medication effects and medical advice. Plan a progressive exercise plan around the client's energy level and lifestyle. Be alert for complaints of adverse effects like dizziness or photosensitivity reactions.

10.	When working with a client who has an injection site(s), skin application, or implanted medication delivery device:

- be very careful about hygiene when assessing or treating the site

- identify the exact location; determine the boundaries and route of any implanted device

- assess the affected tissue thoroughly before treating; do not treat if there are signs of infection or irritation

- exercise appropriate precautions for treatment and hydrotherapy as discussed above

- work outside a 4-6 inch radius of skin patches and implanted devices

1.	*Compendium of Pharmaceutical Specialties*, 28th ed., Canadian Pharmaceutical Association, Ottawa, 1993, pp. 1200-1201

2.	Linde, B., "Dissociation of Insulin Absorption and Blood Flow During Massage of a Subcutaneous Injection Site," *Diabetes Care*, 9(6): 570-574, November/December 1986

3.	Soni, S.D., et al., "Plasma Levels of Fluphenazine Decanoate, Effects of Site Injection, Massage and Muscle Activity," *British Journal of Psychiatry*, 153: 382-384, 1988

4.	Ueda, W., et al., "Effect of Gentle Massage on Regression of Sensory Analgesia During Epidural Block," *Anaesthesia and Analgesia*, 76: 783-5, 1993

5.	*The Mirkin Report*, Bethesda MD, www.wdn.com/mirkin

6.	Manor, D. & Sadeh, M., "Muscle Fiber Necrosis Induced by Intramuscular Injection of Drugs," *British Journal of Experimental Pathology*, (4): 457-462, August 1989

Commonly Prescribed Medications and Treatment Planning

CHAPTER 6

Drugs for Managing Pain and Inflammation

The most commonly consumed over-the-counter (OTC) preparations in the United States are the non-steroidal anti-inflammatory drugs (NSAIDs). This drug group includes aspirin and acetaminophen. In Canada, 1996 sales of OTC analgesics are estimated to have been $197.8 million; in 1997 this figure jumped to $215.9 million.[1] Extrapolating to the U.S. market, sales figures of approximately ten times this amount are likely.

The estimated annual cost associated with toxicity of NSAIDs (excluding non-upper gastrointestinal hemorrhage and hepatotoxicity) is about $1.35 billion![2] These drugs are also very frequently taken alongside of other medications. For example, a 1998 study estimated that almost 20 million patients and 12% of the U.S. population aged 60 or more are taking NSAIDs and antihypertensive medications concurrently.[3] Given the widespread use and ease of availability of the NSAIDs, massage therapists will be treating an increasing number of clients who are using these medications for pain and inflammation.

Beyond the volume of over-the-counter sales, prescribed analgesics constitute a very large percentage of North American medication consumption. This chapter will address the following drug classes:

- The Non-Steroidal Anti-Inflammatory Drugs (NSAIDs)
- The Narcotic Analgesics
- Skeletal Muscle Relaxants
- The Corticosteroids

1.   THE NON-STEROIDAL ANTI-INFLAMMATORY DRUGS (NSAIDS)

Drugs belonging to this group are referred to as the non-steroidal anti-inflammatories to differentiate them from the corticosteroids, another group of drugs with anti-inflammatory properties. The primary difference lies in their chemical structures.

Aspirin is the prototype of this group and is used to compare the properties of newer NSAIDs as they are developed. In addition to acetaminophen (Tylenol), examples of common NSAIDs include ibuprofen (Advil), naproxen (Anaprox), and diclofenac (Voltaren).

The NSAIDs are widely used in the management of **mild to moderate** pain and inflammation. Most members of this group demonstrate all of the following properties:

- anti-inflammatory
- analgesic
- antipyretic (fever lowering)
- anticoagulant

Acetaminophen (Tylenol) is something of an exception in that it produces less anti-inflammatory action than the other NSAIDS. Instead, it is widely used for its antipyretic and analgesic properties.

This drug group is very large. Physicians, in choosing which NSAID to prescribe or recommend, consider factors like age and constitution of the patient, drug cost, and the pharmacologic activities most required in the situation.

Uses

The NSAIDs are mainly used in the following conditions:

- inflammatory conditions such as rheumatoid arthritis, tendinitis, bursitis (exception: acetaminophen)
- osteoarthritis
- minor orthopedic/dental surgery, toothache, headaches, sport injuries, etc.
- dysmenorrhea
- more recently, for cardiovascular diseases because of their anticoagulant effect (aspirin is mainly used for this purpose)
- for cough and cold symptoms such as mild fever and body aches (primarily acetaminophen)

Mechanism of Action

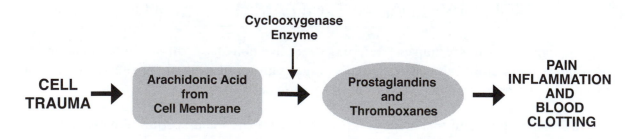

The actions of prostaglandins and thromboxanes contribute to the symptoms of tissue trauma.

Irritated or traumatized cells release arachidonic acid into their tissue interstitia. In the presence of the enzyme cyclooxygenase, arachidonic acid is converted into prostaglandins and thromboxanes. The NSAIDs inhibit the synthesis and actions of prostaglandins and thromboxanes, primarily through impairing cyclooxygenase activity.

There are several types of prostaglandins – the ones involved in the inflammatory response are found in most body tissues. These prostaglandins are produced in high concentrations following any type of cell irritation or trauma. In addition to inflammation, the increased prostaglandin volume is associated with pain creation and with increased smooth muscle contraction in the gastrointestinal, circulatory, and respiratory systems. Through inhibiting the formation of prostaglandins, the NSAIDs reduce the pain and inflammation associated with trauma.

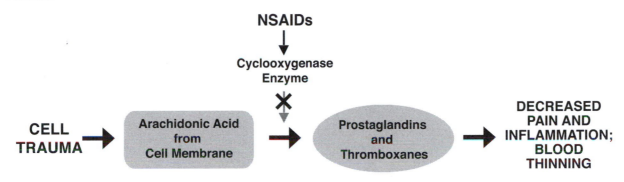

The NSAIDs reduce the formation of prostaglandins and thromboxanes.

Prostaglandins also play an important role in kidney function and protection of the gastric mucosa. This is why NSAID drugs, which inhibit prostaglandin formation and function in varying degrees (aspirin being particularly effective in this respect), are associated with side effects such as gastric irritation and various forms of kidney dysfunction.

Thromboxanes stimulate platelets to stick together. Persons with high thromboxane (especially thromboxane A2) levels are more predisposed to thrombosis (blood clot formation) and other types of cardiovascular problems.

The NSAIDs, especially aspirin, reduce blood clot formation. While a certain amount of clotting control is good, for example following a stroke (cerebrovascular accident), when the blood does not clot as it should the person may experience more bleeding and bruising than usual. Clients using NSAIDs will be at risk for increased bruising following deep tissue work.

2.   THE NARCOTIC ANALGESICS

The narcotic analgesics are also referred to as the opiates. The prototype of this group of drugs is morphine; other members are drugs such as hydrocodone, pethidine, and codeine.

The narcotic analgesics are used to manage **moderate to severe** pain, both short-term and chronic.

Because these drugs have the potential to produce physical dependence, they are classified as controlled substances and require a doctor's prescription. Codeine is an exception. Preparations containing high codeine doses are classified as controlled substances; however, many OTC pain medications combine acetaminophen or aspirin with small doses of codeine.

Uses

The narcotic analgesics are typically used for the management of pain from:

- debilitating injuries
- severe fractures
- major surgery
- terminal diseases
- chronic conditions characterized by severe pain

Mechanism of Action

Although the exact mechanism of action of these drugs is still being examined, they mimic the activities of the endorphins, enkephalins, and dynorphins, which are the body's own naturally produced opiates.

Opioid receptors are found on cells in the brain, spinal cord, and peripheral nerves. Several different types of opioid receptors have being discovered, each having specific effects. The narcotic analgesics are believed to act at these sites to alter cellular functions associated with pain perception and transmission.

Research suggests several possible mechanisms, including:

- **altering the flow of calcium and potassium in and out of the cell**

Calcium and potassium are important elements needed for proper neuronal function, that is, transmission and conduction of impulses across synapses and along neurons within CNS tracts and peripheral nerves. When the normal activities of these substances are interrupted the transmission of pain signals can also be interrupted.

- **affecting cellular second messenger systems**

Second messenger systems are intracellular mechanisms of communication that can either stimulate or inhibit certain cell functions. The opioid drugs are believed to inhibit the formation of intracellular second messengers such as cyclic adenosine monophosphate, a possible mechanism of altering pain transmission.

When acting within the central nervous system, the narcotic analgesics:

- reduce the patient's perception of pain
- alter the reaction and emotional response to pain
- produce sleep
- depress the respiratory, vasomotor, and cough reflex centers

  (codeine is often used as a cough suppressant because of this property)

When acting on the peripheral nervous system, the narcotic analgesics affect sensory neurons at the site of injury/inflammation to produce an analgesic effect. They also directly influence the smooth muscle cells of the gastrointestinal tract to decrease peristaltic motility and increase the tone of the intestinal sphincters. (These effects can be useful for managing diarrhea, but often result in constipation.)

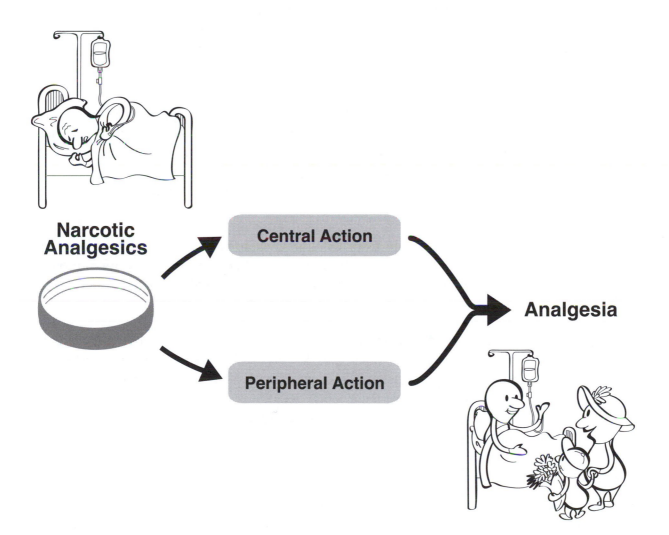

3.   SKELETAL MUSCLE RELAXANTS

The skeletal muscle relaxants are used to reduce muscle tone, primarily to manage muscle spasm and spasticity. These two terms are often used quite loosely and therefore require more detailed explanation.

Muscle Spasm

As a response to trauma, muscles will often 'go into spasm' to protect themselves and traumatized local tissues against further insult. This is sometimes referred to as muscle splinting. A spasm is characterized by an abnormally high increase in muscle tone. The result is usually pain, decreased range of motion, and even inflammation of affected joints.

Spasms can also occur when muscle stretch receptors (the muscle spindles) react strongly to an unexpected stretch, for example inadvertently stepping off a curb or missing a step. The muscle spindle reflexes generate alpha motor neuron signals to the overstretched muscle to produce sudden forceful contraction.

Spasms can also result from intrinsic factors such as electrolyte imbalance.

Spasticity

Spasticity, which is caused by injury or insult to the central nervous system, reflects a loss of inhibitory input on normal muscle tone from either supraspinal or spinal centers. Normal muscle tone requires balancing of ascending excitatory signals from the peripheral nerves and descending inhibitory signals from the central nervous system. These inputs are balanced in the ventral horn of the spinal cord where the alpha motor neuron cell bodies are located.

Spasticity is usually caused when brain or spinal cord areas responsible for voluntary movement are harmed. CNS damage from conditions such as multiple sclerosis, cerebral palsy, spinal cord injuries, and stroke can affect the normal control of muscle tone through impairing descending inhibitory signals from the brain and spinal cord to the peripheral reflexes.

Signs and symptoms associated with spasticity include hypertonicity (increased muscle tone including spasm), clonus (a series of rapid muscle contractions), exaggerated deep tendon reflexes, reflex spillover effects where motor responses 'spread' to other body parts, scissoring (involuntary crossing of the legs), and fixed joints. Gait, movement, and speech are usually compromised. Spasticity can vary in degree from mild muscle stiffness to severe, painful, and uncontrollable spasms.

Uses

The skeletal muscle relaxants are subdivided into two general groups, distinguishing those that act within the central nervous system from those whose responses are produced primarily in the periphery.

Centrally acting skeletal muscle relaxants (acting on the CNS) are mainly used to inhibit painful muscle hypertonicity related to soft tissue injury or inflammation.

The **peripherally acting** skeletal muscle relaxants have two primary uses:

- in the management of spasticity, where CNS controls are impaired and therefore cannot be utilized effectively to reduce tone

- as an adjunct to general anaesthesia, to prevent muscle spasms and reflex reactions during surgery

Mechanism of Action

The centrally acting muscle relaxants, such as cyclobenzaprine, are believed to depress both sensory and motor impulses at different sites in the brain and at various levels of the spinal cord. This results in decreased muscle tone, and therefore a reduction in painful occurrences like spasm. Other drugs whose mechanisms of action include CNS suppression, for example anti-anxiety medications, can produce similar effects.

The peripherally acting muscle relaxants create their effects through functioning within the muscle tissue or at the neuromuscular junction to reduce tone. This group includes two main categories:

- drugs that directly influence the skeletal muscle cell, like Dantrolene

- drugs that act at the neuromuscular junction, such as succinyl-choline

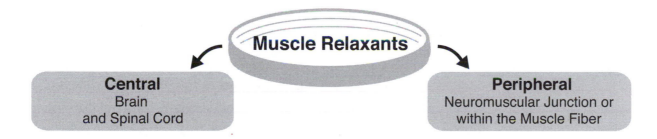

Dantrolene is believed to act on the sarcoplasmic reticulum of the muscle cell to block calcium channels. Calcium ion binding with actin and myosin fibers is necessary for muscle contraction to occur. When a drug like Dantrolene can impair this calcium ion binding, the contractile ability of the muscle is reduced. This type of effect does not rely on neural input.

Dantrolene is primarily used to manage spasticity. It is not recommended for 'ordinary' muscle spasm situations. In therapeutic doses its activities are limited to skeletal muscle, with no action observed in the heart or smooth muscle structures.

Drugs such as succinyl-choline act at the neuromuscular junction (where the alpha motor neuron signal makes contact with the muscle cell membrane) to inhibit the normal activities of the neurotransmitter acetylcholine. Acetylcholine is released from the motor neuron to stimulate the muscle cell. Drugs that suppress acetylcholine can create temporary flaccid paralysis in the body's muscles.

4.   THE CORTICOSTEROIDS

The adrenal glands are primarily responsible for producing the two types of adrenocorticosteroids, namely the mineralocorticoids and the glucocorticoids. The mineralocorticoids, for example aldosterone, play an important role in fluid and electrolyte balance. The glucocorticoids, such as cortisol, have several functions including exercising controls on glucose metabolism, inflammation, and the immune response.

This section will focus on the uses and actions of the synthetically produced glucocorticoids. These drugs are referred to as the corticosteroids. They are among the most widely used in medicine, and are available in forms including tablets, liquids, topical creams and ointments, aerosol sprays, eye/ear drops, and injections.

Uses

The corticosteroids do not actually cure any disease or disorder. Instead, they reduce associated immune or inflammatory responses, providing a more comfortable, less painful lifestyle for the patient.

Corticosteroids are utilized in either **physiologic** or **pharmacologic** (supraphysiologic) doses. Physiologic doses are relatively small and are taken to replace the body's daily production of cortisol. This can be necessary for some adrenal gland disorders, for example Addison's Disease.

When administered in pharmacologic doses, which are much higher, the corticosteroids mimic the actions of naturally produced cortisol to produce anti-inflammatory and immunosuppressant effects. Medically supervised short-term use (1 to 3 weeks) of corticosteroids in pharmacologic doses is usually well tolerated with minimal side effects. However, more long-term use can lead to disruption of adrenal gland functions and an increased likelihood of undesired effects.

The corticosteroids are used in the medical management of:

- autoimmune disorders, for example rheumatoid arthritis and systemic lupus erythematosus

- arthritic and degenerative joint disorders such as ankylosing spondylitis

- non-arthritic conditions like tendinitis and bursitis

- allergic disorders like rhinitis, atopic or contact dermatitis, anaphylactic reactions, and serum sickness (a hypersensitivity reaction that may occur after antiserum administration or in reaction to certain drug therapies)

- dermatological disorders such as psoriasis, seborrheic dermatitis, and alopecia

- gastrointestinal diseases, for example ulcerative colitis, chronic hepatitis, and inflammatory bowel disease

- respiratory disorders like asthma, emphysema, and pulmonary tuberculosis

- transplanted tissue rejection reactions

Therapists should have an appreciation of the widespread use of this group of drugs and make sure to ascertain why any given client is using a corticosteroid medication.

Mechanism of Action

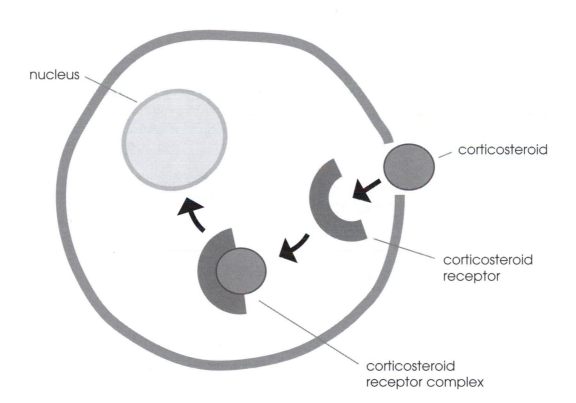

The corticosteroids are believed to act directly on the nuclei of cells. On entering a cell, the drug binds to a glucocorticoid receptor in its cytoplasm. The resulting steroid-receptor complex then travels into the cell's nucleus and combines with specific sites to stimulate the transcription of DNA into messenger RNA. Messenger RNA is responsible for protein synthesis. Several types of proteins are produced, for example enzymes, structural proteins, and messengers, all of which affect cellular functions in various ways. The corticosteroids will generate four main categories of effects:

- anti-inflammatory
- immunosuppressant
- catabolic effects on connective tissues
- effects on other cellular functions

Anti-Inflammatory Effects

The corticosteroids reduce the signs and symptoms of inflammation regardless of its cause. They depress production of several inflammatory substances, including prostaglandins, leukotrienes, histamine, and kinins. Corticosteroids also appear to stabilize capillaries (reduce their natural leakiness), and to strengthen the membranes of intracellular organelles to lessen release of their destructive proteolytic enzymes.

Immunosuppressant Effects

The corticosteroids are thought to inhibit migration of leukocytes and macrophages to sites of inflammation, and also to reduce their responsiveness to key chemical mediators like the interferons and interleukins. The quantities of other important immune system cells, including circulating T-lymphocytes, monocytes, and eosinophils, are also reduced. The overall combined effect is a suppressed immune system.

A less reactive immune system can be useful when managing autoimmune conditions or following organ transplant procedures. However, immunosuppression will make a client more susceptible to contracting infectious diseases.

Catabolic Effects on Connective Tissues

Cortisol has the important metabolic function of maintaining blood glucose and liver glycogen levels. To achieve this, it directs the breakdown of body tissue proteins and fats into amino acids and free fatty acids, which in turn undergo gluconeogenesis in the liver. The new glucose is either released into the blood or stored as glycogen.

In pharmacologic doses the corticosteroids have a similar catabolic effect on the connective tissues of the body. Muscles and their tendons, bones, ligaments, joint capsules and articular surfaces, fascial membranes, and blood and lymph vessels can all be broken down. As well, corticosteroids inhibit fibroblast activity, which will result in reduced connective tissue rebuilding and thinning of skin.

Let's look at some examples of how long-term corticosteroid use causes changes to body tissue structures:

- Injections into joints to manage arthritic conditions can damage articular cartilage, leading to further compromise of the joint surfaces.

- Prolonged skin applications can result in sensitivity loss and reduced skin strength and tone.

- Injections into tendons and musculotendinous units to manage inflammation can reduce the sensitivity of golgi tendon organs and muscle spindles to stretch and tension changes, resulting in a tearing or rupture risk.

- Injections into the plantar fascia can promote rupture, as well as secondary pathologies such as tendinitis of the foot muscles.

- Osteoporosis can develop in susceptible individuals.

Effects on Other Cellular Functions

The results of some of the additional ways the corticosteroids can alter cellular functions include:

- increased resorption of sodium and water in the kidneys (promoting edema and increased blood pressure)

- changes in behavior and mood

- inhibited calcium absorption from the gastrointestinal tract, having numerous potential effects on muscle and neuron function, as well as bone health

- impaired osteoblast activity (increases predisposition to osteoporosis)

Therapists should note that all of the effects of the corticosteroids given above, occurring as they do in combination, will often result in slower healing times, and may lead to a poorer quality of tissue resolution or repair. It is important not to make assumptions about 'standard' healing time frames and to recognize that the effects of a corticosteroid medication in reducing pain and inflammation can lead a site to appear less acute than it really is.

SIDE EFFECTS – Drugs for Managing Pain and Inflammation

This table lists the common side effects of the groups of medications discussed in this chapter. Therapists must keep in mind that other side effects may occur, and that reactions will vary in degree and intensity. Always ask clients about incidence and intensity of any side effects experienced. When more than one medication is being taken, whether in the same drug group or not, therapists should appreciate the increased potential for adverse and idiosyncratic effects.

Side Effects	NSAID	NA	MR	CSD
Abdominal Cramps	XX	X		X
Acne				X
Allergic Reactions	XX			
Anorexia	X	X		
Anxiety		X	X	
Blurred Vision	XX			
Blood Dyscrasias	XX			
Bradycardia		X		
Bruising	XXX			XX
Confusion	X		X	
Constipation	XX	X		
Depression	X		X	
Drowsiness	XX	X	X	
Dry Mouth	X		X	
Diarrhea	X			
Dizziness	XX	X	X	
Euphoria		X		
Facial Flushing			X	
Fatigue		X	X	X
Fever			X	
Fractures				X
Gastrointestinal Bleeding	XXX			X
Headaches	XX		X	X
Hepatitis	XXX			
Hiccups			X	
Hip or Shoulder Pain				X
Hypertension	X			X
Hypotension		X		
Increased Appetite				X
Indigestion			X	
Insomnia	X		X	

Side Effects	NSAID	NA	MR	CSD
Libido Changes			X	
Lightheadedness		X	X	X
Loss of Vision			X	
Menstrual Irregularities				X
Mood Changes	X			X
Muscle Weakness				X
Nausea	XX	X	X	X
Osteoporosis				X
Palpitations	XX			
Peptic Ulcers	XXX			X
Peripheral Edema	X			X
Photosensitivity	XX		X	
Poor Wound Healing	XX			XX
Poor Immune Response				X
Postural Hypotension		X	X	
Prolonged Bleeding Time	XXX			XX
Pruritus	X	X	X	
Rashes	XX	X	X	
Respiratory Depression		X		
Restlessness		X		
Sedation		X		
Shortness of Breath	XX			
Sweating			X	
Tachycardia		X	X	
Tendon Injury	X			XX
Thrombophlebitis				X
Tinnitus	XX			
Tremors			X	
Urinary Retention/Frequency	X	X		
Vomiting	XX	X	X	X
Weakness			X	X

NSAID: Non-Steroidal Anti-inflammatories, NA: Narcotic Analgesics, MR: Muscle Relaxants, CSD: Corticosteroids

The main side effect associated with Dantrolene is liver toxicity.

X – tolerable – notify medical practitioner if bothersome

XX – serious – monitor closely and notify medical practitioner

XXX – very serious – seek medical attention

Quick Guide to Case History Taking

Conditions requiring management of pain and inflammatory reactions range from musculoskeletal trauma to chronic systemic disorders. It is important to clarify the reasons for the use of medications addressing pain and inflammation in each client's case.

Questions

1. What is the cause of the client's pain? Was a medical diagnosis made? Musculoskeletal injury, overuse syndrome? Systemic disorder?

2. Is there inflammation? Local or generalized? Current stage of the inflammatory process? Is this a condition involving flare-ups? If yes, how often? Is there a pattern to what causes them?

3. When did the pain and inflammation start? Pain location - have client identify area(s) of discomfort.

4. What is the nature and description of the pain - sharp, shooting, deep, dull, achy? Have the client rate the pain on a pain scale. Does it affect sleep or daily activities?

5. With respect to the pain and/or inflammation, what alleviates it? Makes it worse (specific movement, rest, activity)? How does it respond to touch?

6. Has the condition got better, worse, reached a plateau?

7. What medications are being used to treat the pain and/or inflammation symptoms? Get details of medication type(s) and reason(s) for use. Any problems with medication effects? If yes, have they been medically evaluated?

8. Any use of medication delivery devices? Self-administering injections? Patches? Clarify location(s).

9. What is the general health status of other body systems? Any systemic conditions, e.g. hypertension, diabetes, asthma? If yes, how are they being managed?

10. Any areas of sensory impairment? Where? Known cause?

11. What other therapies (past or present) have being used to address this problem? What was the response?

Observations

1. Gait: is it normal, antalgic? Is there compensatory or protective holding? Does the facial expression indicate pain during walking?

2. Position of comfort during standing and sitting.

3. Ease with which the client removes coat, shoes, etc. Is help required? Is there an obvious decrease in function or range of motion?

4. Signs of injury and/or inflammation: edema, skin color, bruising, abrasions.

5. Compare bilaterally for size and shape, tissue color, edema, heat/coolness, tissue atrophy.

6. Ability of client to focus and communicate effectively during the interview.

Quick Guide to Working with Clients Who Have Pain/Inflammation

1. **Client Position and Comfort:** Because of the nature of the condition and/or medication effects, the client may not be able to reflect accurately on the comfort and safety of delicate body tissues. The practitioner must pay particular attention to position choices and transfers. Swollen tissues need to be well supported and elevated to encourage drainage. Use pillows and other supports to ensure that any vulnerable body parts are not compromised.

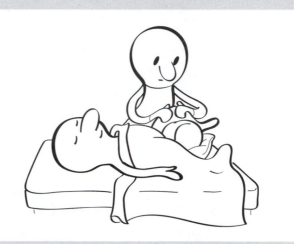

2. **Tissue Health:** Pay particular attention to the health and integrity of the skin and underlying connective tissues. With longstanding or chronic conditions tissues are generally more fragile, tend to have reduced or otherwise altered sensitivity, and can be more easily injured from normal use of manual techniques.

3. **Systemic Health:** Pain and inflammation can be a part of the symptom picture of a systemic disorder. Familiarize yourself with the condition and the specific clinical issues it presents. In the chapters that follow several types of painful and/or inflammatory conditions are addressed, for example respiratory disorders in Chapter 9, cancer in Chapter 11, and HIV/AIDS in Chapter 12. Evaluate the health of systems like the cardiovascular system, which is usually affected by generalized conditions. Pain and inflammation rarely present as unique or independent symptoms – the practitioner must consider the underlying causes and design the treatment approach accordingly.

4. **Effects of Touch:** In most cases professional touch in an appropriately designed treatment approach will help reduce pain. However, it is important to realize that this is not always true. For individuals in severe pain sometimes being touched causes overload and results in more distress and discomfort. This can change from day to day – the practitioner has to be understanding and flexible.

Choice of Techniques

1. In general, client feedback about pain and depth of pressure can be misleading. 'Going deeper,' even if you have the client's encouragement, may result in bruising, worsening the injury, or exacerbating an inflammatory reaction.

2. PROM, effleurage, gentle direct or indirect myofascial therapies, lymphatic drainage, and light reflex techniques like vibrations and stroking and are all effective in treating the edema and muscle tension that often accompany injuries and flare-ups.

Topical Administration of Pain Medications

In an earlier chapter, topical skin applications for relief of muscle and joint pain were discussed. Topical analgesics or counter-irritants like Zostrix and Tiger Balm are often effective in managing pain of the more superficial joints like the knee, hands, and lower back. These preparations act in a variety of ways on the local circulation and superficial nerves to relieve pain and stiffness.

Massage Guidelines – Clients Taking Medications for Pain and Inflammation

General Guidelines

1.   It is important to always keep in mind that the purpose of these medications is to relieve pain. Client feedback, although important to solicit and consider, may be unreliable. The massage therapist must assume more responsibility than is ordinarily the case for determining what treatment approaches are safe and appropriate.

2.   Make sure you are aware of all the medications the client is taking, whether prescription or OTC. Keep in mind that drugs for managing pain and inflammation are addressing symptoms. Especially when the cause is a systemic condition, various other medications may also be employed and will need to be taken into account in treatment planning. Be alert to the fact that multiple medication use can predispose to a higher incidence of adverse effects.

3.   Schedule treatments around medication taking to maximize the accuracy of the client's feedback and to optimize medical stability. These issues are addressed in more detail in Chapter 5.

4.   Nausea and vomiting are potential side effects of all the medication types discussed in this chapter. Such episodes can leave the client feeling weak and fatigued. Postponing the session or giving a shorter, more specific treatment may be required.

5.   Dizziness, drowsiness, and postural hypotension are also common side effects. These can be heightened by massage. Ask your client about post treatment reactions – future treatments may need to be shortened or less intense. Always instruct the client to sit up slowly and stay seated on the massage table for a minute or so before standing up.

6.   Clients taking narcotic analgesics and corticosteroids often experience mood changes and may be less communicative or responsive. The therapist may notice that the client is less cooperative, or seems disinterested in responding in a meaningful or thorough fashion to requests for information or feedback. It can be necessary to exercise a bit more professional assertiveness.

7.   Some clients will experience skin irritations. Ensure proper positioning, and keep in mind that local massage is contraindicated until the reaction has subsided.

8. Topically administered pain and anti-inflammatory medications act in a variety of ways on the local circulation and superficial nerves to relieve pain and stiffness. They tend to compromise local sensation. If on-site work is otherwise appropriate, exercise caution and modify depth of pressure when working on tissues being influenced by such topical applications.

Specific Guidelines

1. Non-Steroidal Anti-Inflammatory Drugs (NSAIDs)

These drugs have both analgesic and anticoagulant properties. Clients may be unable to give accurate feedback about technique pressures and will be more susceptible to bruising if treated too aggressively.

Be alert to complaints of gastrointestinal pain and discomfort. The NSAIDs can cause ulcers and GI tract bleeding, both of which can become life threatening if not addressed medically. If the client has been diagnosed and is being treated for GI side effects, abdominal massage and hydrotherapy are contraindicated until the condition has resolved.

2. Muscle Relaxants and Narcotic Analgesics

The muscle relaxants and narcotic analgesics depress neural responses. Stretching techniques should be avoided or applied cautiously because sensory feedback from muscular stretch and tension receptors may be compromised. On palpation, the muscles whose role it is to protect themselves and their local tissues will feel hypotonic.

Constipation is a common side effect of the narcotic analgesics. The decreased intestinal motility is not greatly influenced by massage techniques. Prolonged constipation or bowel restriction must be carefully monitored by the physician.

3. Corticosteroids

The catabolic activity of the corticosteroids, especially with long-term use, can impair tissue strength, resilience, and sensitivity. Skin integrity may be reduced. The body tissues are more easily damaged by pressure and stretch. Massage techniques that place stress on the muscles, bones, and joints of the body must be avoided or modified. Examples include rib springing, heavy tapotement, and passive overpressure. Remember that healing times may be longer than expected, and tissue repair may not be of the best quality. Be particularly careful with clients who are at risk for developing osteoporosis, like postmenopausal women and the elderly.

The corticosteroids have immunosuppressant effects and can make a client more susceptible to infection or communicable 'bugs.' Hygienic routines become especially important. As well, the practitioner should be alert to the need to reschedule such clients' appointments when personally unwell.

Hydrotherapy Guidelines

Before making treatment decisions, always inquire carefully about areas of sensory impairment, everyday hydrotherapy tolerance, and any restrictions the doctor has placed on hydrotherapy use. Small 'trial' applications can be useful. In general, local treatments to specific body areas using modified temperatures are suggested. Always check with the client to see if there were any post-treatment adverse effects.

Keep in mind that analgesics can modify a client's perception of when an application temperature is too hot or too cold for tissue safety.

With use of drugs that depress the CNS, like the skeletal muscle relaxants and narcotic analgesics, systemic hydrotherapy treatments such as saunas, whirlpool baths, herbal baths, and medicated steams are not recommended. The effects of the medications in combination with generalized vasodilation from the treatment can lead to adverse effects like dizziness, fainting, disorientation, confusion, and edema of the extremities.

Be observant with clients who are taking corticosteroids long-term. Get a sense of their general constitutional strength and the acuity of their reactions to hot and cold.

Prolonged topical use of corticosteroids not only causes changes in skin sensitivity but can also affect the reaction of the local blood vessels to hot and cold. Cutaneous blood vessels may spasm when exposed to even mild temperature differences.

Exercise Recommendation

Medications for pain and inflammation can 'take the pain away,' and clients can easily overwork vulnerable tissues, either inadvertently or hoping that doing more will help them get better sooner. A progressive exercise plan should be implemented starting with low resistance, fewer repetitions, and careful monitoring of reactions and progress.

Some people experience photosensitivity reactions from NSAID and muscle relaxant use. When outdoors such clients should be well clothed and perform exercise activities in shaded areas or during cooler times of the day.

Clients taking NSAIDs and narcotic analgesics may experience shortness of breath during exercise. If this occurs the client should be medically evaluated. Exercise frequency, intensity, and duration will probably need to be modified.

1. Nielsen A.C., Market Track, supplied by the Nonprescription Drug Manufacturers Ass'n of Canada

2. McGoldrick, M.D. & Bailie, G.R., "Nonnarcotic Analgesics: Prevalence and Estimated Economic Impact of Toxicities," *Annals of Pharmacotherapy*, 31(2): 221-7, February 1997

3. Ruoff, G.E., "The Impact of Nonsteroidal Drugs on Hypertension: Alternative Analgesics for Patients at Risk," *Clinical Therapeutics*, 20(3): 376-87, May/June 1998

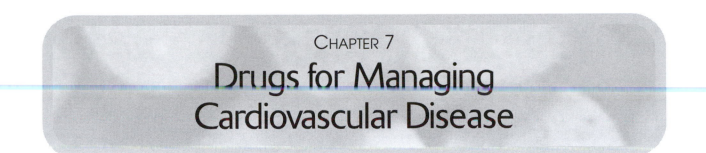

CHAPTER 7
Drugs for Managing Cardiovascular Disease

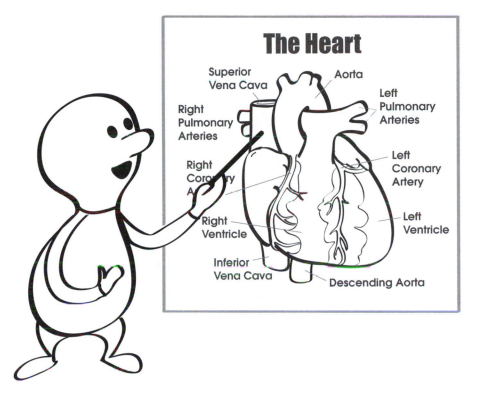

The American Heart Association in their Heart and Stroke Statistical Update (*Economic Cost of Cardiovascular Diseases in 2001*) projects the cost of cardiovascular diseases and stroke in the United States in 2001 will be $298.2 billion. This figure includes health expenditures (direct costs for physicians and other professionals, hospital and nursing home services, medications, home care, and so on) and lost productivity resulting from morbidity and mortality.

Cardiovascular disease is so prevalent that it is estimated about 20% of adult North Americans will develop a cardiovascular condition, most commonly hypertension, atherosclerosis, angina pectoris, heart attack, cardiac dysrhythmia, or stroke. Someone has a stroke every 53 seconds in the United States; a fatal stroke occurs every 3.3 minutes. Cardiovascular disease is usually managed with exercise, diet, stress management and other healthy lifestyle changes, and with a variety of pharmacological and surgical approaches. Massage therapists are frequently in the position of working with clients who are taking one or more medications for a cardiovascular disorder.

COMMON CARDIOVASCULAR CONDITIONS

Atherosclerosis

A condition involving build-up of fatty plaques, called atheromas, inside artery walls. The atheromas project into the blood vessel lumen, reducing flow to supplied tissues and causing blood turbulence that predisposes to thrombus development.

Thrombus

A clot-like plug formed when platelets are activated inside a blood vessel or heart chamber. A thrombus consists of aggregated platelets, fibrin strands, and entrapped red blood cells. The process of thrombus formation is called thrombosis.

Embolus

An embolus is material circulating in the bloodstream that should not be there, for example, a bone chip or nitrogen bubble. The most common emboli are thrombus pieces (thromboemboli) that have detached from their sites of origin. An embolism occurs when an embolus blocks a smaller blood vessel, killing the tissue the vessel supplies.

Angina Pectoris

Episodes of heart pain (intermittent ischemic attacks) brought on by stress and exertion. The cause is reduced blood flow to the heart muscle due to narrowing of its supplying artery(ies), usually because of atherosclerosis but sometimes as a result of vasospasm or constrictive scarring. When the metabolic demand of the myocardial cells exceeds what their compromised circulation can deliver, lactic acid accumulates and pain results.

Myocardial Infarction (MI)

Death of a section of the heart wall because the supplying coronary artery has become blocked or has ruptured; in lay language referred to as a heart attack. Occlusion is most commonly caused by a thrombus developing at an atheroma site.

Hypertension

Chronically elevated blood pressure. Can be idiopathic or as a result of a known cause.

Cardiac Dysrhythmia

Irregular heart beat. There are many possible causes, including conduction system malfunctions, electrolyte imbalances, scar tissue in the heart wall, and drug reactions.

Cerebrovascular Accident (CVA)

Death of brain tissue as a result of blockage or rupture of a supplying artery; commonly called a stroke. Hypertension and atherosclerosis complicated by thrombosis are the usual causes.

Transient Ischemic Attack (TIA)

Intermittent ischemic attacks affecting the brain tissue. As with angina pectoris in the heart, they occur when the lumen of a supplying artery is narrowed due to atherosclerosis, scarring, or vasospasm. In the brain these attacks can produce any number of symptoms, for example blurred vision, slurred speech, muscle weakness, loss of sensation, etc., depending on which tissue area is affected. TIAs are often stroke precursors.

Congestive Heart Failure (CHF)

Weakness of the heart as a pump. The heart struggles to overcome peripheral resistance and supply enough blood to the tissues. Blood pressure and heart rate are elevated. Acute CHF is an emergency situation; chronic CHF is a slow progressive diminishment of the heart's strength and effectiveness.

Blood Pressure, Heart Rate, and Cardiovascular Disease

The role of the cardiovascular system is to provide the body's cells with nutrients and to remove their metabolic wastes efficiently. It is very sensitive to tissue requirements and, when healthy, adapts accurately to minute shifts in metabolic need.

The response of the cardiovascular system to heightened tissue demand is to:

- increase the blood pressure

- increase the heart rate

- redirect blood flow to prioritize tissues under stress

These are normal responses designed to enhance delivery of cellular requirements. They are effective in handling higher demand situations. However, they are intended to be short-term immediate reactions that subside with the end of the stressor. Let's take a closer look at blood pressure and heart rate, since these are the mechanisms most influenced by cardiovascular drug therapies.

- **blood pressure**

Blood pressure is a measure of the relationship between cardiac output and the total peripheral resistance. Cardiac output (CO), defined as the volume of blood the heart pumps per minute, reflects the pumping strength of the heart, its rate and rhythm, and the volume of blood returned to the heart (venous return). The total peripheral resistance (TPR) is a summation of all the elements that create resistance to the flow of blood, therefore determining how hard the heart has to pump to overcome them. The most important factor is blood vessel diameters in the systemic and pulmonary circulations. The volume and viscosity of the blood also affect TPR.

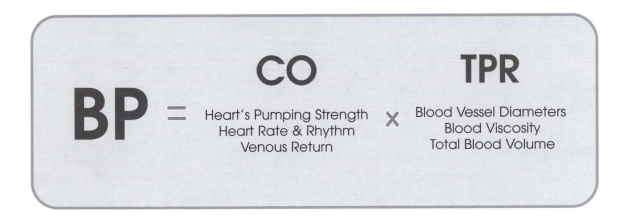

When blood pressure is consistently elevated above normal levels concerns arise because of the stress this places on the heart and vasculature. Monitoring blood pressure is one of the diagnostic tools routinely used to assess the health of the cardiovascular system.

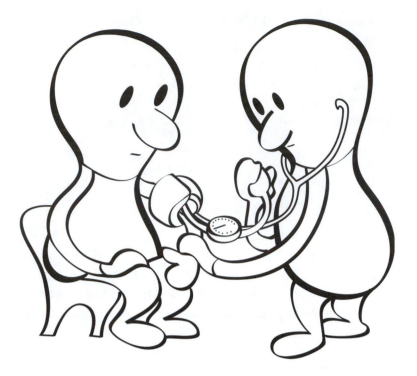

Chronic blood pressure elevation, called hypertension, is generally defined in an adult as a systolic pressure of 140 or higher and/or a diastolic pressure of 90 or higher on more than one visit within two weeks. (Infants and children can also develop hypertension, but different diagnostic criteria are used.)

Hypertension is classified into two categories:

- primary or idiopathic hypertension, which accounts for 90-95% of cases
- secondary hypertension (caused by another diagnosed condition), which accounts for 5-10% of cases

The diagnosis of hypertension is almost always an indication of increasing cardiovascular stress. When high blood pressure is lowered, the stress and work of the heart are reduced and circulatory efficiency is improved.

- **heart rate**

The average normal resting heart rate is 70-72 beats per minute. There is considerable range in what is considered normal, however; children have faster resting heart rates, and elite athletes generally have much slower ones.

As the heart is asked to do more work, it starts to beat faster. Within physiologic limits, the faster the heart beats, the more blood it can pump. Signaled by the sympathetic nervous system, the healthy heart reacts to added demands by increasing both the rate and force of its pumping action. Again, this is intended to be a short-term response.

The heart muscle is nourished between contractions, so a rapid heart rate reduces the time frame in which the heart wall itself can be perfused with fresh blood. If the heart rate is chronically elevated, eventually the tissue is weakened. The weaker heart will tend to beat faster to compensate, creating an unfortunate cycle characteristic of progressive heart failure.

An elevated heart rate does not necessarily indicate stronger myocardial contractions; in fact, the opposite is often true.

Medications and Cardiovascular Disease

When drugs are used in the treatment of cardiovascular disorders they are often directed at managing blood pressure or strengthening heart function, or both. As well, medications are often employed to prevent or control factors that may lead to blood vessel narrowing or blockage.

The medications commonly prescribed for cardiovascular conditions are grouped into categories of drugs that:

- improve heart function
- increase blood vessel diameter
- alter blood coagulation mechanisms
- reduce blood volume
- lower blood lipid levels (reduce blood vessel blockage)

It is important to keep in mind that the drugs we will be discussing in this chapter are often used in combination with each other – individuals with cardiovascular problems are frequently taking several medications.

1.   DRUGS THAT IMPROVE HEART FUNCTION

This grouping includes two main drug classes:

- the beta blockers (beta-adrenergic blocking drugs)
- the cardiac glycosides

Beta Blockers

The beta blocker medications are among the most widely used in the management of cardiovascular diseases. They act on microscopic areas called beta-adrenergic receptors (beta receptors) located on the surface of the heart. These receptors are normally activated when sympathetic neurotransmitters like adrenaline and norepinephrine are released during stress. When the beta receptors are stimulated in this manner, the heart's rate and force of contraction are increased as part of the 'fright, flight, and fight' survival response. Added work from the heart is a necessary part of being able to act quickly to avert an accident or escape from a risky situation.

Concern arises when there is unnecessary or chronic sympathetic stimulation of the beta receptors. The natural rate and rhythm of the heart can be adversely affected and it can begin to weaken from overstress and reduced perfusion.

Uses

The beta blockers are primarily used in the management of:

- hypertension, angina pectoris, and dysrhythmia

- vascular headaches (migraines)

- anxiety and tremors

Commonly prescribed betablocker medications include: propranolol (Inderal), nadolol (Corgard), metoprolol (Lopressor), and timolol (Blocadren).

Mechanism of Action

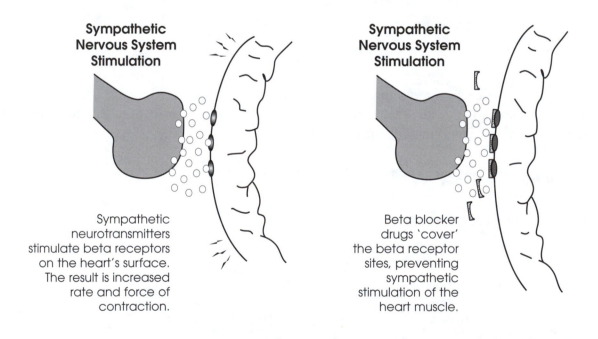

Sympathetic Nervous System Stimulation

Sympathetic neurotransmitters stimulate beta receptors on the heart's surface. The result is increased rate and force of contraction.

Sympathetic Nervous System Stimulation

Beta blocker drugs 'cover' the beta receptor sites, preventing sympathetic stimulation of the heart muscle.

The beta blocker drugs compete with sympathetic neurotransmitters for the beta receptor sites on the heart, 'occupying' and blocking them. By preventing sympathetic stimulation of these sites, the beta blockers relieve cardiac stress by slowing myocardial contractions and improving their rhythmicity. The beta blockers also seem to have a systemic effect of reducing blood vessel constriction, thereby assisting in lowering the blood pressure and easing stress on the heart.

Beta receptors are located in many organs, including the heart, lungs, liver, and skeletal muscle tissues. Activation of the beta receptors stimulates the formation of the second messenger cyclic AMP, which then either activates or inactivates certain cellular enzymes.

There are two major types of beta receptors, called beta-1 and beta-2. Stimulation of beta-1 receptors usually produces an excitatory effect in the target tissue cells, as is the case with the heart. Beta-2 receptor activation generally results in inhibitory effects; for example, in the lungs stimulation of such sites reduces constriction of bronchial passages.

The discovery of these specific beta receptors led to the development of beta-selective drugs. Early beta blockers were non-selective in nature – they occupied both beta-1 and beta-2 sites. When an individual took one of these beta blockers for a cardiovascular condition, there was a risk of serious respiratory side effects such as precipitating or worsening an asthma attack. This risk is reduced with the newer drugs.

Cardiac Glycosides

Cardiac glycosides are commonly found in plants such as milkweed, lily of the valley, the oleander plant, and foxglove. Medicinal use of these plants for heart conditions dates back at least 3,000 years – the Egyptians, Romans, and early Europeans all used them. Today, the cardiac glycosides are mainly derived from various species of the foxglove plant and include drugs such as digitalis, digitoxin, and digoxin. Collectively these drugs are often referred to as digitalis, and that is how we will refer to them in this section.

Uses

The cardiac glycosides are primarily used for:

- treatment of congestive heart failure
- prophylaxis and treatment of cardiac dysrhythmias

Congestive heart failure (CHF) results when the heart is not pumping effectively to meet the demands of the body tissues. CHF can be an acute situation, such as right ventricular failure due to a pulmonary embolism. This is a life-threatening condition that requires immediate medical intervention and will not be seen by the massage therapist in everyday practice.

However, massage practitioners are more likely to be working with clients with chronic progressive heart failure, the incidence of which is quite high in North America. This type of congestive heart failure is a slower loss of strength and efficiency of the heart that results in structural and physiological changes and eventual death of the myocardial tissues.

Mechanism of Action

The overall effect of the cardiac glycosides is to reduce the workload of the heart by:

- slowing down the heart rate
- increasing the efficiency of the contraction and refilling phases of the cardiac cycle

Although the exact mechanism is still not completely clear, research suggests two main actions of the cardiac glycosides:

- Digitalis produces a positive inotropic effect on the heart (increases the force of myocardial contraction) by altering the normal functioning of the sodium/potassium pump. An electrolyte imbalance is created that causes an influx and release of calcium ions within the myocardial cells.

  Calcium ions are important for normal and efficient cardiovascular function. They play a key role in contraction of the heart wall, in contraction of the muscles of the blood vessels, and in the heart's electrical conduction system. When the normal progress of calcium ions in and out of their cells is altered, the contractile and electrical properties of these structures are affected. Pathways (gates) for the movement of intracellular calcium are regulated by a number of hormonal, electrical, and chemical processes.

  The cardiac glycosides influence this gating activity, elevating intracellular calcium concentrations to trigger biochemical events that result in more forceful contraction. Following myocardial contractions the ventricles are more completely emptied, while on refilling they are more completely filled. These effects aid in improving blood circulation to the body tissues and reducing peripheral edema.

- Digitalis also seems to have an effect on the heart's electrical conductivity mechanisms. The conduction rate of impulses at the atrioventricular (AV) node is reduced and there appears to be more vagus nerve stimulation; these effects decrease the heart's electrical excitability and slow the heart rate.

2.   DRUGS THAT INCREASE BLOOD VESSEL DIAMETER

The drugs discussed in this next section all increase vascular diameters. Although their mechanisms of action differ, their common effect is vasodilation. The purpose is to decrease peripheral resistance and lower blood pressure.

We will look at four categories of commonly prescribed drugs with vasodilation effects:

- the vasodilators
- the calcium channel blockers
- the angiotensin-converting enzyme (ACE) inhibitors
- the alpha receptor drugs

Vasodilators

The 'official' vasodilator medications (those that are actually called the vasodilators) belong to a group of drugs that are chemically related to the nitrates, for example nitroglycerin. The nitrates and their derivatives are available in several forms including sublingual tablets, aerosol sprays, ointments, and skin patches.

Uses

The nitrate family of drugs is used in the management of:

- angina pectoris, acute and chronic
- hypertension
- congestive heart failure

Mechanism of Action

These drugs act directly on the coronary and peripheral blood vessel walls to reduce their tone. They are metabolized to nitrous oxide in the vascular smooth muscle cells. Nitrous oxide is a chemical that exists naturally in the body to help regulate blood vessel contractility. It does so via increasing the concentration of a second messenger called cyclic GMP[1] which produces vasodilation.

It was once believed that the nitrates only dilated the affected vessels of the heart during an angina pectoris attack. Although some coronary vasodilation is observed, the relief produced is mainly due to dilation of the systemic vasculature. This lessens the peripheral resistance and reduces the filling of the ventricles, cutting back quickly on the stress placed on the heart. When used as directed under the tongue for angina attacks, these effects take place within 2-3 minutes.

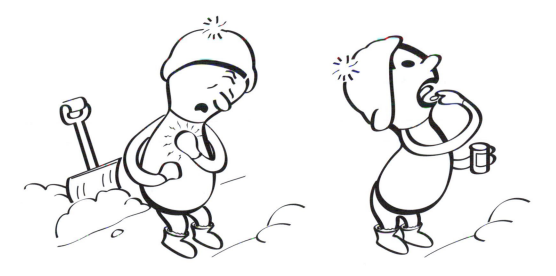

Calcium Channel Blockers

These drugs, used very commonly in treating high blood pressure, also produce their effects by influencing smooth muscle tone in blood vessel walls.

Uses

The calcium channel blockers are widely used in medical practice for:

- hypertension
- tachycardia (rapid heart beat)
- prevention of migraines
- prevention of vascular spasm after brain hemorrhages

Commonly prescribed calcium channel blockers include: Cardizem (Diltiazem), nifedipine (Procardia), and verapamil (Isoptin).

Mechanism of Action

The calcium channel blockers act on the intracellular calcium gates in cardiac and vascular smooth muscle cells to block influx and movement of calcium ions. Their key effects, which work together to reduce stress on the heart, include:

- **vasodilation**

Vasodilation of the coronary blood supply increases blood flow and oxygen to the heart, assisting it to function more effectively. The vasodilation of the peripheral vasculature eases stress on the heart by reducing peripheral resistance and venous return.

- **reduction of the rate and force of cardiac contraction**

Heart muscle tone is reduced. Some members of this drug group also slow down the electrical conductivity of the heart. Overall, myocardial excitability is decreased and the heart functions in a more 'relaxed' manner.

ACE Inhibitors

The ACE inhibitors produce vasodilation by interrupting the activities of one of the enzymes in the renin-angiotensin system.

The Renin-Angiotensin System

The kidneys play a crucial role in long-term blood pressure control. One of the mechanisms involved is the renin-angiotensin system, which acts to increase blood pressure back to normal if it begins to drop.

1. Renin is an enzyme produced mainly in the kidneys and released into the circulation in response to a decrease in blood pressure. Renin acts on the substance angiotensinogen, which is made in the liver and is continuously circulating in the blood, converting it to angiotensin I.

2. Angiotensin I is converted to angiotensin II by an enzyme called angiotensin converting enzyme (ACE).

3. Angiotensin II has very powerful vasoconstrictor properties. When it circulates in the bloodstream generalized vasoconstriction occurs and blood pressure goes up.

Massage Therapy & Medications

The renin-angiotensin system is an intrinsic control mechanism that is very useful in circumstances where the blood pressure is dropping. It functions as a homeostatic response in minor circumstances and as a life-preserving mechanism in more severe situations like shock or illness. However, some people develop elevated levels of circulating renin without any apparent reason. In this scenario, the renin-angiotensin system becomes a factor causing hypertension.

Uses

The ACE inhibitors are commonly used in the management of:

- hypertension
- congestive heart failure

Commonly prescribed medications in this group include: Captopril (Copoten), enalapril (Vasotec), and lisinopril (Zestril).

Mechanism of Action

The ACE inhibitors suppress the function of angiotensin converting enzyme, which converts angiotensin I to angiotensin II. When angiotensin II formation is reduced, its ability to cause vasoconstriction is decreased. A reduction in peripheral resistance results and systemic blood pressure is lowered.

The ACE inhibitors also seem to reduce the release of the adrenal hormone aldosterone, which promotes retention of sodium and water by the kidneys. Aldosterone has the potential to produce hypertensive effects because it can cause an increase in total blood volume. The ACE inhibitor drugs, by decreasing the influence of aldosterone on the kidneys and promoting more excretion of water and sodium, lower the blood volume and help decrease blood pressure.

Alpha Receptor Drugs

Alpha receptors are found in the central nervous system and the smooth muscle of blood vessel walls. They belong to two groups:

- alpha-1 receptors located on vascular smooth muscle cells
- alpha-2 receptors found in synapses in the autonomic nervous system

The alpha receptors respond to the sympathetic neurotransmitters epinephrine and norepinephrine to alter blood vessel tone. Alpha-1 receptor activation has a direct effect on the blood vessels to produce vasoconstriction. When alpha-2 receptors are stimulated there is a decrease in the number of sympathetic impulses leaving the vasomotor center, which results in peripheral vasodilation.

Uses

Drugs that act on the alpha receptors are used in the management of:

- hypertension
- congestive heart failure
- Raynaud's vasospasm

Mechanism of Action

Specialized drugs have been designed that can affect sympathetic activity at the alpha receptor sites to decrease vascular tone:

• by blocking stimulation of alpha-1 receptors in the blood vessels

Drugs that occupy and block the alpha-1 receptor sites against sympathetic stimulation are called the alpha-adrenergic antagonists. Examples include prazosin (Minipress), doxazosin (Cardura), and the ergot alkaloid derivatives.

• by stimulating alpha-2 receptors in the CNS

Medications designed to stimulate alpha-2 receptor sites in the brain are known as adrenergic agonists and include drugs such as clonidine (Catapres) and methyldopa (Aldomet).

In either case, the overall effect is to decrease the sympathetic mediated tone of the vasculature, causing vasodilation and lowering blood pressure by reducing total peripheral resistance.

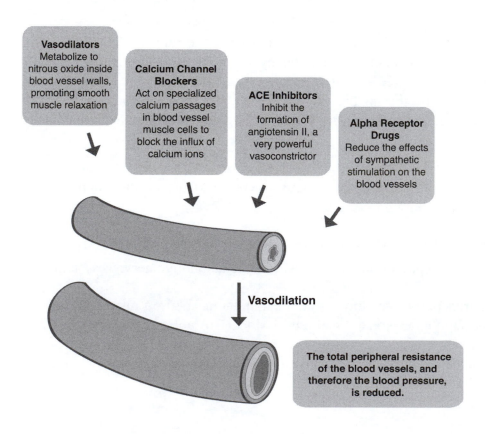

Drugs that increase blood vessel diameter

3. DRUGS THAT ALTER BLOOD COAGULATION MECHANISMS

Blood coagulation is a vital biological function necessary to stop bleeding. Under healthy conditions there is a delicate balance between clot formation and clot breakdown. If clot formation continues unchecked it leads to thrombosis which can obstruct the blood vessel. On the other hand, if clot development is inadequate there is excessive bleeding.

Any factor that causes either too much or too little blood coagulation contributes to cardiovascular stress and disease. Pathological conditions, genetic influences, and the physio-logical changes of aging can all impair blood-clotting mechanisms. Hemophilia is an example of a genetic condition characterized by a defective blood coagulation process – the blood fails to clot and abnormal bleeding occurs. A different example, thrombocytosis, is a condition of various causes characterized by a higher number of circulating platelets. This results in increased blood viscosity, intravascular platelet clumping, and thrombus formation.

This section will focus on drugs that reduce blood clot and thrombus formation, and drugs that are used to 'break up' clots and thrombi.

Drugs used in the treatment of cardiovascular disease to influence blood coagulation processes can be subdivided into three categories:

- anticoagulants (affect blood clotting)
- antithrombotics (inhibit thrombosis by altering how platelets adhere together)
- thrombolytics (break down clots and thrombi that have already formed)

Uses

The anticoagulants, antithrombotics, and thrombolytic drugs are used either alone or in combination with other agents to address:

- deep vein thrombosis
- various thromboembolic and circulatory disorders, including those associated with heart attacks, cardiac and other types of surgery, pulmonary emboli, strokes, and transient ischemic attacks

Mechanism of Action

• anticoagulants

The two most commonly used anticoagulant drugs are the orally administered coumarin derivatives, such as warfarin, and the parenterally administered drug heparin.

Warfarin, which has a similar chemical structure to vitamin K, competes with vitamin K at its active sites in the liver. Vitamin K functions and dependent processes are suppressed, resulting in reduced formation of several of the blood clotting factors. It can take a number of days for the coumarin derivatives to produce their anticoagulant effects.

Vitamin K is necessary for normal blood clotting. It acts as a catalyst during the synthesis of four of the twelve factors in the clotting cascade: II (prothrombin), VII, IX, and X. It also plays a role in the conversion of prothrombin to thrombin; thrombin is needed for the conversion of fibrinogen to fibrin. Fibrin strands form the meshwork of clots and thrombi.

Heparin is only administered by intravenous or subcutaneous injection because it is not absorbed when taken orally. The body has its own natural source of heparin – it is abundant in granules of the mast cells that line the vasculature.

Heparin increases the activity of a substance called antithrombin III, which forms complexes with thrombin. The antithrombin III-thrombin complex inhibits several key enzymes in the blood clotting process. Unlike warfarin, heparin's onset of action is very quick. These two drugs are often used in combination for immediate and longer-term effects in the treatment of venous thrombosis and embolism.

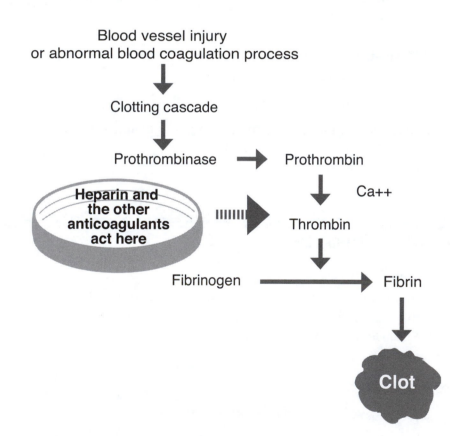

The anticoagulants produce their effects by interfering with the production of fibrin.

- **antithrombotics**

Drugs that prevent or impair platelet aggregation reduce the risk of dangerous thrombus formation. The antithrombotics are anti-platelet drugs. They are used mainly in the prevention of arterial thrombosis, especially in the coronary and cerebral arteries.

Unlike blood clots, which form through a "cascade" of clotting factor processes, thrombi develop as a result of platelet activation. In the presence of the chemical mediator thromboxane A2, platelets clump together (aggregate). Aggregated platelets, entrapped red blood cells, and fibrin are the usual components of thrombi.

Platelets play an important role in controlling bleeding, especially following tissue trauma. However, thrombi can create risky situations if blood vessels are obstructed. Platelets can also be activated by blood vessel inflammation or elements like atheromas that cause blood turbulence.

A drug that is increasingly being used as an antithrombotic agent is aspirin. As discussed previously, aspirin inhibits the formation of thromboxanes. A single dose of aspirin can inhibit platelet aggregation for up to a week. Since platelet life span is 6-10 days, aspirin (or other NSAIDs with similar properties) can inactivate platelets for most or all of their short lifespan.

Another example of an antithrombotic medication is dipyridamole (Persantin), which also inhibits platelet aggregation. It is often used following prosthetic heart valve replacement to prevent thromboembolic complications.

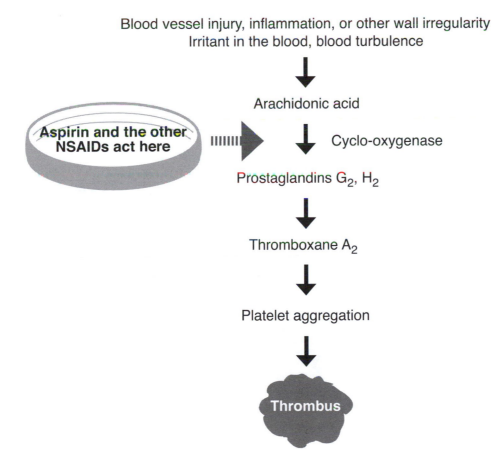

The antithrombotics produce their effects by impeding platelet aggregation.

- **thrombolytics**

The thrombolytic drugs promote disintegration of clots and thrombi that have already formed. This process depends on the presence of plasmin, which is the enzyme responsible for breaking down fibrin mesh. Any drug or agent that increases plasmin formation and/or activity has the potential to be used to promote clot and thrombus dissolution.

Streptokinase is an example of a drug in this class. It is an enzyme that combines with plasminogen (the inactive precursor of plasmin) to form a plasminogen-streptokinase complex. This complex facilitates plasmin formation.

Another substance that is successfully used pharmacologically as a thrombolytic agent is a commercial form of the naturally occurring compound tissue plasminogen activator (tPA). During normal clot breakdown plasminogen is activated by the body's own tPA. DNA technology has recently made tPA available as a thrombolytic drug.

The thrombolytics are used in the treatment of arterial and venous thrombi, after strokes and heart attacks, and to clear IV catheters and other such devices.

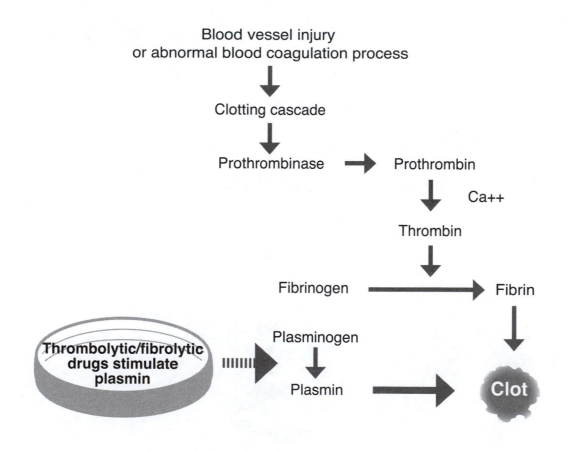

The thrombolytic drugs produce their effects by stimulating increased plasmin formation.

4. DRUGS THAT REDUCE BLOOD VOLUME (THE DIURETICS)

The diuretics are usually the first drugs of choice in the pharmacological management of hypertension and heart disease. They are generally well tolerated and are safely used in combination with other cardiovascular drugs. The main action of the diuretics is to increase the formation of urine. They do this through direct action on various parts of the kidney tubule system. An increase in urine volume leads to a reduction in total blood volume, which is another avenue for decreasing blood pressure.

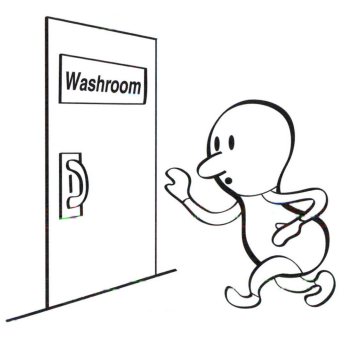

The diuretics discussed in this section are classified into three groups:

- the thiazide diuretics
- the loop diuretics
- the potassium sparing diuretics

Uses

The diuretics are used in the management of:

- primary hypertension
- edema due to congestive heart failure, liver disease
- pulmonary edema
- diabetes insipidus

Mechanism of Action

The diuretics act at different sites in the kidney nephrons to increase urine volume.

- **thiazide diuretics (e.g. Diuril)**

These drugs act at the distal and convoluted tubules to block sodium and chloride ion resorption. When more of these ions are allowed to pass into the urine, via osmosis more water goes with them. There is an associated increased loss of potassium ions, which can cause muscle and nerve dysfunction side effects like cramping and cardiac dysrhythmias.

- **loop diuretics (e.g. Lasix)**

The loop diuretics act primarily on the ascending loop of Henle to selectively inhibit the resorption of chloride ions. With increased loss of chloride ions into the renal tubules there is an accompanying removal of sodium ions and water. Associated potassium loss can be quite high when taking these drugs.

- **potassium sparing diuretics (e.g. Aldactone)**

These drugs act on the distal renal tubules. They inhibit the cellular pump that facilitates elimination of potassium and resorption of sodium. The hormone aldosterone controls this pump. The result is increased sodium and water excretion with conservation of potassium ions.

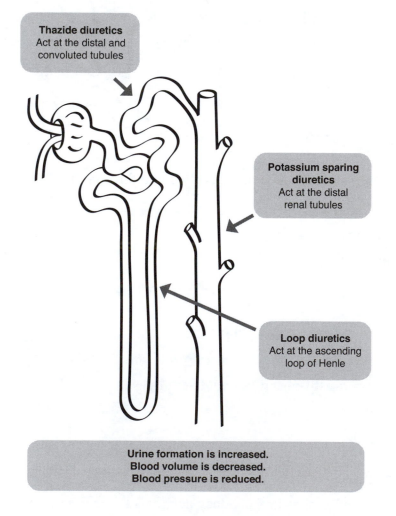

Drugs that reduce blood volume

5.   DRUGS THAT LOWER BLOOD LIPID LEVELS

The lipid lowering drugs (LLDs) are used to manage hyperlipidemia, which is defined as an abnormally elevated plasma lipoprotein level and is considered a key risk factor for developing atherosclerosis.

Hyperlipidemia is classified as either:

- primary (due to genetic/familial tendencies)
- secondary (caused by high dietary fat, especially saturated fats, and poor lifestyle)

The relationship between elevated plasma lipoproteins, in particular cholesterol, and coronary heart disease is well established. An estimated fifty-two million Americans need to comply with dietary changes to establish adequate plasma lipoprotein levels, and almost thirteen million require drug therapy.[2]

The main lipids (fat-like substances) transported in the blood are triglycerides and cholesterol. Under normal healthy conditions they both have important biological functions. Triglycerides are the primary form of fat in the body. They play a key role in supplying calories or body energy. Cholesterol is involved in many cellular functions including formation of cell membranes and hormone production.

Types of Lipoproteins

Lipoproteins are classified according to their density (weight).

1. **Chylomicrons:** Containing about 90% triglycerides by weight, chylomicrons are very large. The fats in the food we eat are digested by the intestines to form chylomicrons which are transported via the lymphatic system into the blood.

2. **Very Low Density Lipoproteins (VLDLs):** VLDLs are comprised of about 60% triglycerides by weight. Unlike the triglycerides of the chylomicrons that come from ingested food, these are made in the liver from endogenous carbohydrate stores. Triglycerides are unable to directly penetrate cells like muscle fibers and fat cells. When they require an energy source, these cells produce an enzyme (lipoprotein lipase) that breaks VLDLs down into fatty acids and glycerol which are able to enter the cell.

3. **Low Density Lipoproteins (LDLs):** These lipoproteins contain about 50% cholesterol and 5% triglycerides. LDLs are the remnants of VLDLs. The liver produces about 70% of the body's cholesterol and most cells can synthesize their own; however if they require additional amounts they produce receptors on their cell membranes for LDL. When an LDL combines with a cell receptor it is taken into the cell and degraded. When the cell has enough cholesterol it stops creating receptors.

4. **High Density Lipoproteins (HDLs):** HDLs consist of 5% triglycerides and 20% cholesterols. They are considered the 'good guys' for several reasons. They take cholesterol from tissue cells to the liver. The liver either breaks down the cholesterol into bile salts or excretes it into the bile. HDLs also seem to inhibit cellular uptake of LDLs, and may discourage aggregation of platelets. The higher the HDL levels the less cholesterol in the bloodstream.

These lipids do not circulate freely in the blood – they bind with protein molecules to form lipoprotein complexes. Excess volumes of these complexes in the bloodstream promote atherosclerosis development.

When pharmaceuticals are employed to manage hyperlipidemia, their overall purpose is to reduce cholesterol and triglyceride concentrations in the plasma. The drugs used for this purpose fall into four main groups:

- the bile acid sequestrants
- nicotinic acid (niacin)
- the fibric acid derivatives
- HMG Co A reductase inhibitors

Drug Group	Mechanism of Action	Comments
Bile Acid Sequestrants Drugs belonging to this group include Questran, LoCholest, and Colestid. Used for managing elevated LDL levels.	These drugs are not absorbed from the GI tract. They bind with bile acid to form an insoluble complex excreted in the feces. This increases the liver's utilization of cholesterol to make bile acids.	The first choice for treating elevated LDL and cholesterol levels.[3] Maximum effects occur after about one month.
Nicotinic Acid (Niacin) Brand names include Niacor, Niaspan, and Nicolar. Used to lower plasma levels of both LDLs and VLDLs.	Niacin is believed to decrease activity of the enzyme triglyceride lipase. This inhibits formation of VLDLs, and in turn LDLs.	The oldest lipid lowering drug. Produces a marked decrease in triglyceride and LDL levels and an increase in HDLs.
Fibric Acid Derivatives Drugs belonging to this group include Atromid-S, Lopid, and Tricor. Used primarily to treat high triglyceride levels.	These drugs activate the enzyme lipoprotein lipase, and may also interfere with the production and release of VLDLs by the liver.	Can reduce triglycerides by up to 45% while increasing HDLs.
HMG Co A Reductase Inhibitors Also known as the statins, these drugs are the most commonly prescribed in the U.S. Brand names include Lipitor, Baycol, Lescol, Mevacor, Pravachol, and Zocor. Used for treating elevated LDL levels.	These drugs inhibit the enzyme 3-hydroxyl-3-methyl-glutaryl coenzyme A, which is important for the synthesis of cholesterol in the liver. They also increase the number of hepatic LDL receptors. The overall effect is a reduction in LDL plasma levels.	LDL plasma levels decrease within two weeks of starting therapy. These drugs have an excellent safety and side effect profile.

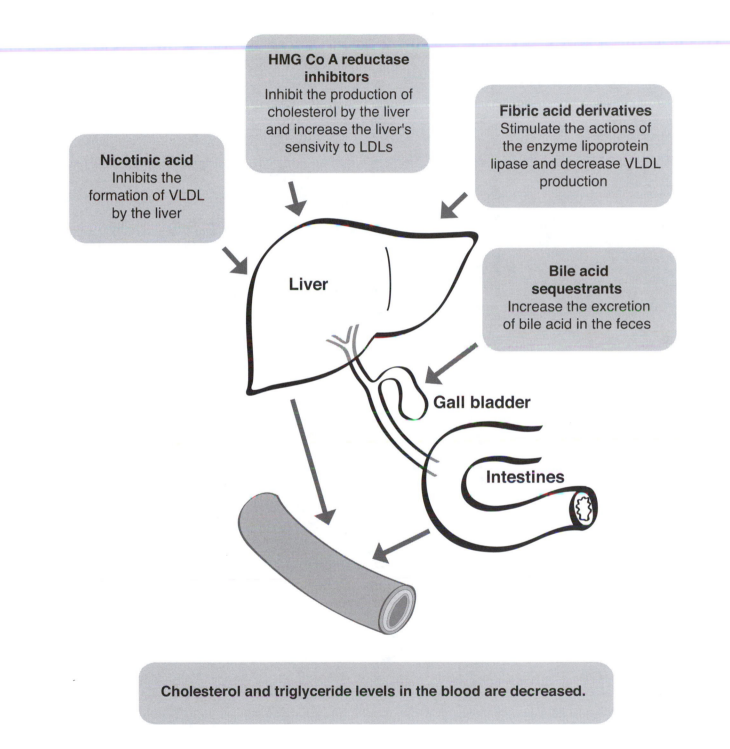

HMG Co A reductase inhibitors
Inhibit the production of cholesterol by the liver and increase the liver's sensivity to LDLs

Fibric acid derivatives
Stimulate the actions of the enzyme lipoprotein lipase and decrease VLDL production

Nicotinic acid
Inhibits the formation of VLDL by the liver

Bile acid sequestrants
Increase the excretion of bile acid in the feces

Liver

Gall bladder

Intestines

Cholesterol and triglyceride levels in the blood are decreased.

Drugs that lower blood lipid levels

SIDE EFFECTS – Drugs for Managing Cardiovascular Disease

This table lists the common side effects of the groups of medications discussed in this chapter. Therapists must keep in mind that other side effects may occur, and that reactions will vary in degree and intensity. Always ask clients about incidence and intensity of any side effects experienced. When more than one medication is being taken, whether in the same drug group or not, therapists should appreciate the increased potential for adverse and idiosyncratic effects.

Side Effects	BB	AC	CCB	ACE	DIU	VD	CG	LLD	ARD
Abdominal Cramps	X	X			X		XX	XX	X
Acne								X	
Allergic Reactions	XXX		XXX				XX	X	X
Anorexia		X					XX	X	
Anemia								XX	
Angina								XXX	
Anxiety	XX		XX	X					X
Appetite Changes					X		XX	XX	
Arthritis								X	
Back Pain	XXX	XXX			XXX				
Blurred Vision	X		XXX	X	XX	XXX	XX	X	X
Blood Dyscrasias	XX	XX		XXX	XXX			X	
Bradycardia	XX		XXX						
Breathing Difficulty	XXX		XXX		XXX			XX	
Bruising	X	XX						XX	
Bursitis								X	
Chest Pains	XXX		XXX	XXX	X			XX	
Cold Extremities	XXX								
Confusion	XXX				X		X	X	X
Constipation	X	X						XX	X
Cough		XX		XX					
Cramps		X			XX			XX	X
Cyanosis						XXX			
Deafness								XX	
Depression	XXX		X				X	X	X
Dreams	X							X	X
Drowsiness	X		XX				X	X	
Dry Eyes	X			X				X	
Dry Mouth	X		X	XXX	XX	XXX		X	X
Diarrhea	XX			X	XX		XX		X
Dizziness	XX	X	XX	XX		X	X	XX	XX
Facial Flushing						XX		XXX	
Fatigue	X		XX	X				X	X
Fever	X	XX	X	X		XXX		XX	
G.I. Bleeding or Pain					XXX	X		XX	XX
Gout								X	
Hallucinations	XX						X		
Headaches	X	XX	X	X	X	XX	X		XX
Hearing Loss								XX	
Hematuria		XXX							
Hepatitis		XXX							
Hyperglycemia					XXX			XX	X
Hypertension								XX	XX
Hypotension	XX		XXX	XXX		XX	XX	XX	

Side Effects	BB	AC	CCB	ACE	DIU	VD	CG	LLD	ARD
Increased Appetite								X	
Insomnia	XX		X	XX				XX	X
Irregular Heartbeat							XX	XX	
Joint Pain	XXX		XXX	XXX	XXX			XX	X
Kidney Dysfunction		XXX		XXX				XX	
Libido Changes	XX		X	X	X			X	X
Lightheadedness			X			X		X	X
Liver Dysfunction					XXX			XX	
Loss of Hearing					XXX			XX	
Loss of Taste				X				X	X
Loss of Vision							XX		
Mood Changes				XXX	XX			X	
Muscle Weakness	X			XX			XX	XXX	X
Nausea	X	X	X	XX	XX	X	XX	X	X
Nasal Stuffiness	X								X
Nosebleeds								XX	XX
Palpitations	X		X					X	XX
Paresthesia	XX		X	XX				XX	
Peripheral Edema	XXX		XX	XXX		XX		X	XX
Photosensitivity			X	X	X			XX	
Postural Hypotension					X	XX		XXX	XX
Prolonged Bleeding Time		XXX							
Pruritus								X	
Rashes	XXX	X	X	XXX		XXX			X
Restlessness						X			X
Shortness of Breath	X					XXX		XX	
Sore Throat	XX	XX		X					
Sweating	X				X	X		X	
Tachycardia	X		XXX			XXX			X
Tendon Injury								XX	
Thirst				XX	XX				
Tinnitus			X	XX	XXX			X	X
Tiredness	X	XX	X	X	XX				
Tremors	X								
Urinary Frequency									X
Vertigo	X				X				X
Vomiting	XX			XX	XX		XX	X	X
Weakness	XX	XX	X		XX	XXX	X		X
Weak Pulse				XXX	XX				
Weight Gain								X	

BB: Beta Blockers, AC: Anticoagulants, CCB: Calcium Channel Blockers, ACE: Angiotensin Converting Enzyme Inhibitor, DIU: Diuretics, VD: Vasodilators, CG: Cardiac Glycosides, LLD: Lipid Lowering Drugs, ARD: Alpha Receptor Drugs

X – tolerable – notify medical practitioner if bothersome

XX – serious – monitor closely and notify medical practitioner

XXX – very serious – seek medical attention

NOTE: Clients using an anticoagulant medication must pay particular attention to any incidence of unexplained bleeding. Signs and symptoms that require immediate attention include: nosebleeds, unusual bruising, blood in the stools or urine, unusually heavy or unexpected menstrual flow, bleeding from the gums, coughing up blood, joint pain/stiffness/swelling, and abdominal pain or swelling.

Quick Guide to CV System Case History Taking

The cardiovascular system is responsible for ensuring that each cell of the body has an adequate supply of oxygen and nutrients, and that metabolites are properly removed. It is important to keep in mind that when the health of the cardiovascular system is compromised all tissues and systems of the body can be affected in one way or another. Similarly, pathologies of other body systems often cause cardiovascular stress.

Questions

1. Identify the cardiovascular disorder(s) for which the client is being treated. Time frame since diagnosis? Progression of the condition?

2. How is the condition managed? Is it stabilized? Medications, diet, exercise regimen, herbal remedies, etc? Get medication specifics. If nitroglycerine is being used, in what form? If tablets, where does the client keep them in case they are needed? If a patch, location?

3. Has there been any medical emergency? If so, what (heart attack, stroke) and when? How was it managed? Any heart surgery? Ongoing complications from any of these?

4. When was the last visit to the medical practitioner? Any recent developments related to the condition? Was the blood pressure taken? What was it? How does it compare to the previous reading? Have stress tests been done? What were the results?

5. Any other systemic conditions: asthma, diabetes, autoimmune, etc.? How managed?

6. Have any restrictions been placed on exercise or hydrotherapy?

7. Circulatory problems, esp. cold hand or feet? Cyanosis? Slower healing times for cuts or injuries? Any numbness?

8. Any shortness of breath? When does it happen? How much stress or exertion is involved? Experiencing shortness of breath in any particular positions, e.g. lying flat?

9. In the event of a medical problem (for example an angina attack) while receiving a treatment, what is the procedure?

Observations

1. Bruising: Note the extent and color. Inquire about how it happened.

2. Varicosities: Bilateral? How torturous or distended are the veins? How resilient is the skin above them?

3. Peripheral edema: Bilateral? Is it pitted? Color and texture of the local tissues?

4. Breathing difficulties: Is the client out of breath? How much exertion was involved?

It is good clinical practice to take blood pressure and pulse readings for clients with cardiovascular system challenges. Monitor especially for unexpected changes that may need medical evaluation, and responses to massage or hydrotherapy treatment.

Quick Guide to Working with Clients Who Have Compromised CV Systems

Client Positioning

- Clients are often asked to begin a massage treatment in the prone position as a matter of routine. For the client with a compromised cardiovascular system this may not be the best position; in fact with moderate/severe high blood pressure or recent heart surgery it may never be appropriate to place the client prone. Ask about how the client sleeps and what positions will work best for the treatment. Use lots of pillows to enhance comfort. Be prepared to treat in modified supine, sidelying, or seated positions.

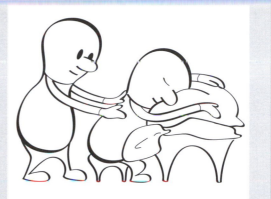

- For clients who have edema, especially of the extremities, ensure that affected areas are well supported and elevate in a manner that promotes natural lymphatic and circulatory flow. However, too much elevation can be stressful on a weakened heart because it increases venous return. For clients with a diagnosis of moderate/severe CHF, do not elevate the feet above the level of the heart.

- Pay particular attention to client position if there is: a recent cardiac surgery, very high blood pressure, an implanted device (e.g. pacemaker or catheter), a medicated patch.

Choice of Techniques

- In general, have a strong focus on relaxing and soothing techniques. The goal is to reduce sympathetic activation, TPR, and the workload of the heart.

- Avoid or modify treatment elements that could activate a sympathetic nervous system response, for example heavy tapotement, deep tissue work, trigger point release, or other potentially painful techniques. Make sure the client is warm enough, and is not caught off guard by anything you are doing.

- Designing the treatment with limb work first helps reduce peripheral resistance.

- Effleurage and petrissage can have potent effects on the circulatory system, especially long strokes that maximize venous return. Smaller segmental techniques like wringing and muscle squeezing increase local circulation without causing as much blood flow back to the heart.

- Avoid excessive elevation or large scale range of motion work when the client has a significantly weakened heart – both can substantially increase venous return.

- When a client has edema, promoting lymphatic drainage can be helpful, but the scale of drainage work needs to be modified with the cardiovascularly challenged client. The lymphatic system empties into the circulatory system and increases blood volume.

- When a client has atherosclerosis or any other condition that predisposes toward thrombosis, depth of technique should automatically be modified. Any known thrombus sites are contraindicated for massage.

- If unsure about the efficacy of your planned approach to treatment, consult with the attending physician.

General Guidelines

1. Make sure you know all the medications being used and why, including OTCs like aspirin. Since clients with cardiovascular disorders are often taking multiple medications affecting various body systems, ask about adverse effects. Research the drugs being taken to see if any of the client's complaints may be related to drug effects.

2. Consider the possibility that massage may destabilize a client with a more severe cardiovascular condition. Timing of massage therapy in relation to medication use, for example if the client has angina pectoris or cardiac dysrhythmias, may be important.

3. Postural hypotension, dizziness, and lightheadedness can occur when using the drugs discussed in this chapter. The client is likely to feel dizzy with fast movements, especially getting up right after a massage. Instruct the client to sit up slowly and wait for a few seconds before getting off the table.

4. Check for injection sites, medicated patches, topical preparation use, and implanted devices. There are cardiovascular medications that are delivered by all these routes. Review the guidelines laid out in Chapter 5.

Specific Guidelines

1. Drugs that Affect Heart Function

The use of beta blockers can precipitate breathing difficulties, chest pains, and abnormal heart rate and rhythm. These symptoms vary in intensity from person to person. They should be carefully monitored medically. Take the client's blood pressure every treatment and pay special attention to any significant symptom changes.

Cold extremities, peripheral edema, paresthesias, and joint pain are common betablocker side effects. Be alert for tissue fragility and decreased sensitivity – when present adjust your depth of technique. Client feedback may not be reliable.

It is estimated that about 25% of people taking digitalis experience some form of toxicity. Therapists should be alert to complaints of gastrointestinal irritation, visual disturbances, confusion, and cardiac abnormalities such as abnormal heart rate or rhythm. If not managed quickly these reactions can become life threatening.

2. Drugs that Increase Blood Vessel Diameter

Kidney disorders, peripheral edema, changes in heart function, and hypotension episodes can occur to varying degrees with this group of drugs. These effects increase the workload of the heart and predispose the client to more serious CV complaints. Check the blood pressure on an ongoing basis and adapt your client positioning and treatment approach as appropriate.

- **ACE Inhibitors** cause some individuals to develop a dry continuous cough within the first several weeks of therapy. Lying in the supine position can make the situation worse by aggravating coughing episodes.[4] Keep some water handy, and consider treating the client in a semi-seated position.

- **Calcium Channel Blockers and Other Vasodilators** can cause swollen, tired feet and ankles. These clients may be at risk for developing deep venous thrombi. Be alert to complaints of persistent pain and cramps. Be prepared to refer these clients to the physician.

- **Nitroglycerine Patches and Ointment** may produce an itchy feeling at the site of application. Do not remove the patch or advise the client to wipe off the ointment. If a rash appears around the patch avoid massaging the affected skin and advise the client to report it to the physician.

3.   Drugs that Alter Blood Coagulation

Clients taking any of the drugs in this group will be predisposed to bruising if treated aggressively. Deep massage techniques such as muscle stripping, cross fiber frictions, and deep kneading techniques are not recommended.

Complaints of low back pain may be related to a concurrent kidney dysfunction. Assess for signs and symptoms of musculoskeletal involvement. If negative, propose follow up medical evaluation.

4.   Drugs that Reduce Blood Volume

Clients taking diuretics may complain of pain, muscle weakness, and cramping/spasms. These can be signs of electrolyte imbalance. Stretching and strengthening procedures must be automatically modified. Heart palpitations may also be related to loss of electrolytes like potassium. These symptoms suggest a need for electrolyte replacement or re-balancing; if the client's M.D. is not aware of them, referral for evaluation is important.

Diuretic use can precipitate occurrences of hyperglycemia. Hyperglycemia signs and symptoms are outlined in Chapter 8. This is a situation that needs to be medically assessed and stabilized.

5.   Lipid Lowering Drugs

Musculoskeletal, cardiac, blood, nervous, gastrointestinal, and metabolic disorders can all occur with use of members of this drug group. Familiarize yourself with the side effect profile of the drug used. Pay attention to chest pain, joint pain, muscle weakness, easy bruising, hearing loss or changes, and changes in blood pressure. Such symptoms should be addressed medically.

Hydrotherapy Guidelines

Always confirm that there are no medically prescribed temperature restrictions, which are common with cardiovascular conditions and cardiovascular drugs like the beta blockers and the vasodilator group. Inquire about daily bath or shower temperatures that are well tolerated.

The drugs discussed in this section will all tend to affect responses of the heart and blood vessels, in one way or another, to temperature changes. The client with a cardiovascular condition is always more at risk for experiencing adverse reactions to hydrotherapy. Begin with the mildest applications and progressively increase the hydrotherapy stimulus, monitoring the client's responses carefully. Local applications are more likely to be appropriate than systemic ones like saunas, medicated steams, and whirlpools. Be watchful for signs of adverse reactions to hydrotherapy. Blood pressure and pulse readings should be taken at the start and end of treatments.

Keep in mind that if the client is experiencing paresthesias, reactions to temperatures will likely be altered.

Exercise Recommendation

The sympathetic response of the heart and blood vessels to exercise requirements will be compromised if the client is taking drugs like the beta blockers or alpha receptor drugs. An aggressive exercise regime puts the client at risk for developing adverse reactions such as abnormal heart rhythm and palpitations.

Ways in which the client's medications may interact with the heating effect from exercise should also be taken into account.

It is important to keep in mind that drugs that affect electrolyte concentrations like the diuretics will predispose the exercising individual to developing cramps and spasms more easily.

Exercise prescription for the most compromised types of cardiovascular patients is a specialized field beyond the scope of most massage therapists. With disorders such as congestive heart failure, a recent stroke or myocardial infarction, and angina pectoris, and considering the myriad of drugs used to treat them, it is best to work with a health care team that provides the services of a qualified exercise therapist.

1. Saari, J.T., Dahlen, G.M., "Nitric Oxide and Cyclic GMP are Elevated in the Hearts of Copper-Deficient Rats," *Medical Science Research,* 26: 495-497, 1998

2. Shafeer, R.S., Lacivita, C.L., "Choosing Drug Therapy for Patients with Hyperlipidemia," *American Academy of Family Physicians*, 61: 3371-82, 2000

3. "Management of Hyperlipidlemia," Website: www.humana.com/providers/guidelines/hyperlip.asp

4. U.S. Pharmacopeial Convention, Inc., *Drug Information for the Health Care Professional (USP DI)*, 12th ed., pg. 257, Maryland, 1992

CHAPTER 8
Medications for
Managing Diabetes Mellitus

Diabetes is the world's most common metabolic disease. In 1997 the direct and indirect costs involved in managing diabetes in the United States totaled an estimated $98 billion. Approximately 6 percent of the U.S. population has diabetes, and it is the fourth leading cause of death. Being diabetic can reduce life expectancy by as much as 30 percent.

Diabetes mellitus is primarily a disorder of carbohydrate metabolism. Since carbohydrates are a basic energy source for cellular activities, such a fundamental problem can give rise to dysfunctions in virtually every body system. Some of the many complications of diabetes include nerve damage (diabetic neuropathy), blood vessel damage (diabetic microangiopathy), skin ulceration, cardiovascular disorders, kidney disease, blindness, seizures, and amputations of limbs and digits.

The central issue in diabetes mellitus is a problem with the body's production and/or utilization of the hormone insulin. One of insulin's key responsibilities is to move glucose from the blood into body cells. It is also an anabolic hormone, playing an important role in tissue growth and repair.

Diabetes is characterized by elevated levels of glucose in the blood (hyperglycemia) and in the urine (glycosuria). The causes of diabetes mellitus are still under investigation. Several types have being identified and are presented in the table on the following page.

The pancreas, the organ involved in diabetes, consists of specialized clusters of cells called the islets of Langerhans. These cells produce and secrete several hormones. There are three specialized cell types found among the islet cells, each of which is responsible for a specific hormone:

- A or alpha cells (glucagon)
- B or beta cells – the most abundant (insulin)
- D or delta cells (somatostatin)

Insulin and glucagon are both involved in regulating blood glucose levels. Insulin facilitates the movement of glucose out of the bloodstream into the peripheral tissues, including muscles. It therefore decreases blood glucose. Glucagon, an antagonist to insulin, increases blood glucose concentration. Somatostatin plays a role in gastrointestinal absorption and may also assist in coordinating insulin and glucagon functions.

Types of Diabetes Mellitus	Characteristics and Risk Factors
Type 1 Diabetes Previously called insulin-dependent diabetes mellitus (IDDM) or juvenile-onset diabetes	Accounts for 5-10% of diagnosed cases of diabetes; usually onsets during childhood. The pancreas ceases to produce insulin, so proper management involves the administration of exogenous insulin. Risk factors for its development, either separately or in combination, include genetic inheritance, autoimmune dysfunction, viral infections, and environmental factors.
Type 2 Diabetes Also referred to as non-insulin dependent diabetes mellitus (NIDDM) or adult-onset diabetes	Accounts for 90-95% of diagnosed cases. The pancreas still produces insulin, but its output may be decreased or the insulin quality may be deficient. Alternatively, the insulin may be normal but peripheral cellular membrane resistance may have developed, meaning that body cell insulin receptors malfunction (for example, in obesity). Another possibility is that the insulin is being broken down before it completes its physiologic function. Usually occurs in adults; is typically managed with diet and lifestyle changes and pharmaceuticals, sometimes with insulin supplementation. Risk factors include older age, overweight, family history of diabetes, prior history of gestational diabetes, impaired glucose tolerance, physical inactivity, and race/ethnicity (e.g. blacks and natives have higher risk inheritance factors).
Gestational Diabetes Develops during pregnancy but recedes when the pregnancy is over	Develops in 2-5% of all pregnancies. Women who are obese or have a family history of diabetes are at higher risk. Women who have gestational diabetes are more likely to develop Type 2 diabetes in later life. Managed with insulin and/or oral medications.
Diabetes From Other Causes	1-2% of diabetes diagnoses. Linked to specific genetic syndromes, surgery, drug effects, malnutrition, infections, and other illnesses. Managed with insulin and/or oral medications.

Management of Diabetes Mellitus

The management of diabetes typically involves:

- use of insulin and/or oral medications
- compliance with a specialized diet that controls sugars and fats
- stress and anxiety management (they increase levels of circulating glucose)
- developing a medically approved exercise plan
- regular medical monitoring
- ideally, becoming a member of a diabetes care support group

In this chapter, we will focus primarily on the pharmaceuticals used in diabetes treatment.

Medication Use in Diabetes

The pharmaceuticals used in managing diabetes include:

- parenteral insulin

- oral hypoglycemic medications

- a combination of insulin and hypoglycemic drugs

1.   INSULIN

Insulin is normally released from the pancreas B cells in response to an increased volume of glucose in the circulating blood, most notably after meals. The insulin stimulates delivery of the glucose into cells, where it is important for numerous metabolic processes. A normal blood glucose level is 80-90 mg per 100 ml of blood. The aim of administering exogenous insulin is to normalize levels of blood glucose in the diabetic.

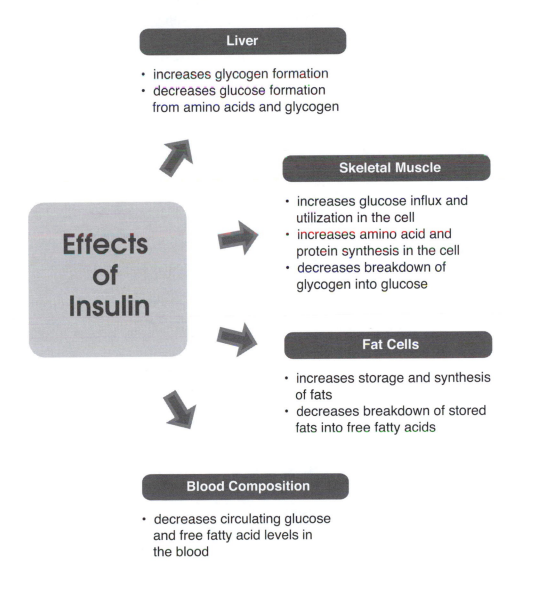

Liver
- increases glycogen formation
- decreases glucose formation from amino acids and glycogen

Effects of Insulin

Skeletal Muscle
- increases glucose influx and utilization in the cell
- increases amino acid and protein synthesis in the cell
- decreases breakdown of glycogen into glucose

Fat Cells
- increases storage and synthesis of fats
- decreases breakdown of stored fats into free fatty acids

Blood Composition
- decreases circulating glucose and free fatty acid levels in the blood

Insulin is utilized in the management of the following:

- type 1 diabetes

- type 2 diabetes when exercise, diet, and oral hypoglycemic drugs are not effective in controlling blood glucose levels

- gestational diabetes

- pregnancy in type 2 diabetic women

- individuals who become diabetic with severe infections, or following surgery or injury, or as a result of medication use (e.g. the corticosteroids can have this effect)

Types of Insulin

There are a number of sources of insulin. Beef and pork insulin are derived by extraction from the pancreas of the animal. These have been widely used but cause allergic reactions in some people. Synthetic forms have also been available for some years. A form of insulin has recently been bioengineered that is identical to human insulin.

Pharmaceutical insulin types vary in their onset, peak, and duration of action, and as such are used for specific effects.

Type of Insulin	Properties and Uses
Rapid Acting or Short Acting	Brand names include Humulin R and Novolin Toronto. Following injection, absorption occurs after 30-60 minutes; peak action occurs after 2-3 hours. Duration of action varies between 6 to 8 hours. Best taken 30-45 minutes before meals.
Intermediate Acting	Brand names include Lente and NPH. Following injection, absorption occurs after 3-4 hours; peak effects occur after 7-9 hours. Duration of action varies between 12 to 16 hours. Best use is at bedtime to control glucose levels the next morning. When taken in the morning peak effects occur in the afternoon.
Very Rapid Acting	Brand names include Humalog (insulin Lispro). Following injection, absorption is very rapid; peak action occurs about 30 minutes later. Best used before meals to control postprandial glucose rise. Can be used as a substitute for short acting insulin.
Long Acting	Brand names include UltraLenta. Following injection, absorption is slow; peak effects occur 10-12 hours later. Variable duration of action lasting between 16 and 18 hours. Mainly used as a substitute for intermediate acting insulin to decrease hypoglycemia incidence during the night.

Insulin duration and activity times vary greatly among different insulin types, from individual to individual, from circumstance to circumstance, and even for the same person using different injection sites. Therapists are encouraged to learn more about the particular insulin type(s) a client is using, the dosing method, and how they react to their insulin.

Insulin Administration

Insulin is protein based – if taken orally it is broken down in the gastrointestinal tract. It is therefore administered by injection, usually subcutaneously.

Insulin can be administered in two different ways:

- multiple daily injections (MDI)
- via an insulin pump

Injection

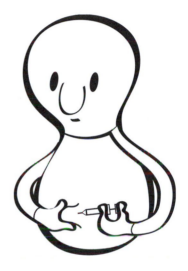

Managing blood glucose levels may require up to four insulin injections per day. Clients are generally well trained in self-injecting insulin in various body locations. Commonly used areas include:

- the abdominal wall
- the lateral arm
- around the waist and hips
- the thigh

Insulin injected in the vicinity of the stomach appears to have the fastest onset of action. The second fastest is usually the arm, while slowest onset occurs with injection into the thigh. The diabetic individual will consistently vary injection sites.

External Insulin Pumps

Insulin pumps are a more recent innovation. They are devices that can be programmed to automatically release insulin. Worn externally and connected to the diabetic's bloodstream via a catheter, design improvements are making insulin pumps increasingly smaller and more user friendly. If the ultimate goal is to create a device that monitors the diabetic's blood glucose and releases insulin exactly as needed (as occurs in the non-diabetic body) insulin pumps have not yet reached this level. However, many diabetic experts now favor insulin pump use over injections. The pump offers the user many benefits:

- more ease in carrying and administering insulin
- better blood sugar control
- flexibility of eating patterns
- easier involvement in sports and other activities

The insulin pump consists of several parts:

- a reservoir for insulin

- a small battery-operated pump

- a computer chip that controls insulin delivery

Current versions of the pump are about the size of a deck of cards, weigh about three ounces, and can be worn on a belt or in a pocket. Connected to the pump is a flexible plastic tube ending with a needle that is inserted just under the skin in the abdominal area. The site of the needle is changed every few days. The user programs the pump to deliver a steady amount (basal dose) of insulin throughout the day. Following meals or at other times when blood glucose may be high, the user can direct the pump to release a 'bolus' dose of insulin.

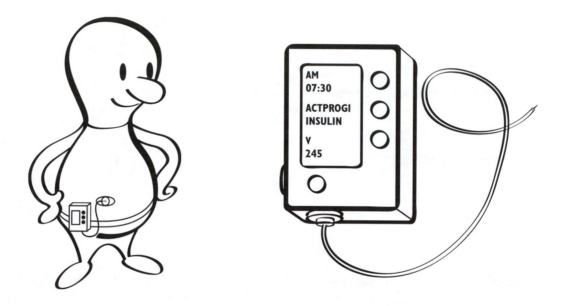

Other devices that are being tested or are in early use for administering insulin include:

- **insulin pens**

Insulin pens are a convenient and discreet way to carry insulin. A fine, short needle sits at the tip of the pen. The user turns a dial to select the desired dose of insulin and presses a plunger to deliver it. The pens are either disposable or have replacement insulin cartridges.

- **insulin jet injectors**

These injectors use a high-pressure air mechanism instead of a needle to send a fine spray of insulin through the skin.

- **implantable insulin pumps**

These pumps are surgically implanted and can be programmed to deliver insulin in a basal dose or continuously as needed. Researchers hope that in the future this type of pump will become a device that can react in the same ways the body would to increased blood glucose.

- **insulin inhalers**

These are under development and close to clinical trials. The insulin used is specially manufactured so it can be sprayed and inhaled into the mouth. The insulin coats the mouth, throat, and tongue and is rapidly absorbed into the bloodstream. These inhalers will most likely be used in combination with other methods of insulin administration.

Mechanism of Action

Insulin influences the production, transport, and utilization of glucose. Specific insulin receptors are located on cell membrane surfaces. When insulin binds to an insulin receptor a series of intracellular biochemical reactions takes place to produce a number of biological compounds. It is believed that these compounds act as second messengers within the cell to facilitate its uptake of glucose and/or to increase its glucose storage. Several intracellular substances including calcium are necessary to these processes.

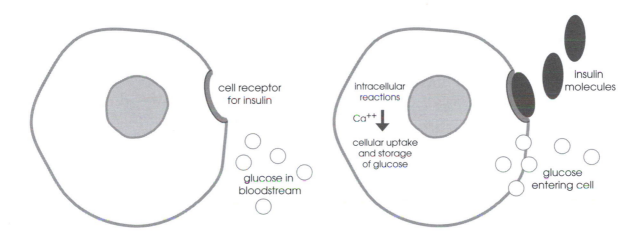

Most cells have insulin receptors on their cell membranes and are referred to as insulin dependent cells. However, brain and kidney cells, red blood cells, and those lining the GI tract do not have insulin receptors. They are able to absorb and use glucose in the absence of insulin stimulation. These cells are referred to as insulin independent cells.

2. ORAL HYPOGLYCEMIC DRUGS

The oral hypoglycemic drugs are used to lower blood glucose levels. They are subdivided into four main categories:

- the sulfonylureas
- the biguanides
- competitive inhibitors of intestinal brush-border alpha-glucosidases
- the thiazolidinediones

Sulfonylureas

The sulphonylureas support insulin release and are only helpful when the person's pancreas is capable of producing insulin. They are commonly prescribed in combination with diet and exercise therapy in the long-term management of type 2 diabetes. They are not effective for type 1 diabetes.

Uses

- type 2 diabetes
- used in conjunction with insulin injections if large amounts of insulin are needed

Commonly prescribed medications in this group include chloropropramide (Diabinese) and glipizide (Glucotrol).

Mechanism of Action

The sulphonylureas promote insulin release from the pancreas. Insulin production is not actually increased, but its secretion from beta cells is. In addition, these drugs appear to enhance the sensitivity of the peripheral tissues to insulin, facilitating glucose uptake into cells. The overall effect is a reduction in blood glucose. Since these drugs increase blood insulin levels, they can potentially precipitate hypoglycemic episodes. This issue will be discussed later in the chapter.

Biguanides

Metformin (Glucophage), a member of this group, has been in use worldwide for the past four decades. It not only lowers blood glucose but also reduces the risk of atherosclerosis development by lowering blood cholesterol and triglyceride levels.

Uses

- managing type 2 diabetes when other drugs are ineffective
- combines well with the sulfonylurea drugs to enhance effects
- for patients who show signs of insulin resistance and are obese

Mechanism of Action

The biguanide drugs use a different method than the sulphonylureas to lower blood glucose. Rather than acting on the pancreas, they target the peripheral tissue cells. Their exact mechanisms of action are still unclear, but they appear to:

- decrease hepatic glucose production
- decrease intestinal absorption of glucose from food sources
- increase peripheral glucose uptake and utilization by improving insulin sensitivity in skeletal muscle and fat cells

Two advantages of this group of drugs are that they do not typically cause hypoglycemia, and they do not promote weight gain. In fact, they are also used to manage some of the complications associated with insulin resistance that are commonly seen with obesity.

> Gastrointestinal distress (stomach upset, cramps, nausea, and vomiting) are common side effects of the biguanide drugs. These types of GI tract activity can lead to increased elimination of vitamin B12. Signs of B12 deficiency include fatigue, depression, easy bruising, skin sensitivity, peripheral neuropathy (numbness and tingling), and loss of appetite.

Alpha-Glucosidase Inhibitors (Starch Blockers)

This class of drugs was first released in the United States in 1995. Their potential for use in combination with the sulfonylureas and biguanides makes them an important addition to the medications available for managing type 2 diabetes.

Uses

- type 2 diabetes

A commonly prescribed example of this group is acarbose (Precose).

Mechanism of Action

These drugs act in the intestines by reversibly inhibiting the alpha-glucosidase enzyme. The role of this enzyme is to break down complex carbohydrates into glucose. Carbohydrate absorption is forced to take place further along the gastrointestinal tract, producing a more gradual and delayed rise in postprandial blood glucose concentration.

Thiazolidinediones (TZDs)

This new class of hypoglycemic drugs first became available in the United States in 1997. An early member of the group, troglitazone, was withdrawn from the market in March 2000 because it was seen to cause severe idiosyncratic liver injuries. Rosiglitazone (Avandia) and pioglitazone (Actos) have been available since 1999 and have safer profiles.

Uses

- type 2 diabetes

Mechanism of Action

Studies suggest that these drugs increase cell membrane sensitivity to insulin and normalize a wide range of metabolic problems associated with insulin resistance.

TZDs act on a specific receptor called the peroxisome proliferator activated receptor gamma (PPAR gamma). PPAR gammas are predominantly found in adipose tissue, macrophages, vascular smooth muscle cells, endothelial cells, and several cancer cell types. These are all target tissues for insulin and when stimulated show increased insulin sensitivity.

Beneficial effects of the TZDs include:

- improved glucose uptake in skeletal muscle, adipose tissue, and hepatocytes
- reduced fasting hyperglycemia and insulinemia
- decreased plasma triglyceride, free fatty acid, and LDL-cholesterol levels
- increased plasma HDL-cholesterol concentrations

Sulfonylureas
- Promote release of insulin from the pancreas
- Increase the sensitivity of peripheral tissue cells to insulin

Biguanides
- Decrease liver glucose production and intestinal absorption of glucose
- Increase peripheral glucose uptake and utilization

Alpha-Glucosidase Inhibitors
- Act in the intestines to inhibit the enzyme alpha-glucosidase
- Delay digestion and absorption of complex carbohydrates

Thiazolidinediones
- Increase glucose uptake in muscle and fat cells and in the liver
- Decrease blood triglyceride, fatty acid, and cholesterol levels

Blood glucose levels are reduced.

Actions of the oral hypoglycemic drugs

SIDE EFFECTS – Drugs for Managing Diabetes

This table lists the common side effects of the groups of medications discussed in this chapter. Therapists must keep in mind that other side effects may occur, and that reactions will vary in degree and intensity. Always ask clients about Incidence and Intensity of any side effects experienced. When more than one medication is being taken, whether in the same drug group or not, therapists should appreciate the increased potential for adverse and idiosyncratic effects.

Side Effects	Insulin	Sulfonylureas	Biguanides	Alpha-glucosidase Inhibitors	TZD
Abdominal Cramps		XX	XX	XX	
Allergic Reactions	XX				
Anemia					X
Blurred Vision		X			
Bloating				XX	
Blood Dyscrasias		XX			
Bruising			XX		
Confusion		X			
Constipation		X			
Drowsiness		X			
Diarrhea		X	XX	XX	
Dizziness		X		XX	
Edema					X
Fatigue		X	XX		
Flatulence				X	
GI Distress		XX	XX		
Headaches					X
*Lipodystrophy/Lipohypertrophy	X				
Liver Dysfunction		XX			XXX**
Hypoglycemia	XXX	XXX			
Metallic Taste			X		
Muscle Weakness		XX			
Nausea			X		
Paresthesia		XX			
Photosensitivity		X			
Rashes	X	XX			
Tinnitus		X			
Tremors		X			
Vertigo		X			
Vit B12 Deficiency			XX		
Vomiting			XX		
Weakness		XX			
Weight Gain					XX
Weight Loss			X		

 * refers to changes in the subcutaneous fat at injection sites
** blood tests to monitor liver function are done frequently

X – tolerable – notify medical practitioner if bothersome

XX – serious – monitor closely and notify medical practitioner

XXX – very serious – seek medical attention

Diabetic Instability Reactions

Diabetics are constantly challenged to find the right balance between insulin and blood glucose. Blood glucose levels that are either too high or too low can cause a number of symptoms, at their worst progressing to life-threatening destabilization. Even though medications are central to diabetes management, their use can also be a factor in diabetic instability episodes.

Hyperglycemia, which is the 'natural' diabetic condition, can jeopardize tissues like the brain whose cells uptake glucose without assistance from insulin and can reach toxic levels if blood glucose becomes too high. Severe hyperglycemia produces a state called **diabetic coma**. Pharmacologically, hyperglycemia can occur from underjudging medication requirements, from using an insulin product that is not a good match for the patient's needs, from missing a dose, or as a medication side effect.

On the other hand, if the diabetic misjudges and uses too much insulin, or does not eat enough to match insulin intake, or takes too much or too powerful an oral hypoglycemic drug, available glucose is mobilized into cells and the blood glucose level can become seriously low. This is called **insulin shock**. It can be difficult to judge doses on a day-to-day basis because, as we will discuss shortly, a number of circumstances can alter the diabetic's pharmaceutical requirements. Insulin shock can also occur as a medication adverse effect.

In severe or untreated diabetic instability crises, loss of conscious, convulsions, and eventual death can occur.

Episodes of diabetic instability can onset rapidly or more slowly. In general, hypoglycemia onsets more quickly and hyperglycemia onsets over a few days. The table below is a quick reference for signs and symptoms of hypo- and hyperglycemia.

HYPOGLYCEMIA (leads to insulin shock)	HYPERGLYCEMIA (leads to diabetic coma)
stomach pains	abdominal pain
hunger	anorexia
nervousness	thirst
shallow breathing	air hunger
pallor and fatigue	shortness of breath
sweating	facial flushing
weakness	polyuria
continuing headaches	headaches
tachycardia	weight loss
unsteady gait	nausea and vomiting
confusion	acetone breath
moist and pale skin	dry and flushed skin
convulsions	constipation
normal eyeballs	soft eyeballs

First Aid for Diabetic Instability Episodes

Since diabetic instability can become life-threatening, it is important to have a good grasp of first aid guidelines. The more the person giving assistance is familiar with the diabetic person, the more tailored the reaction can be. Unless expert, the first aid provider should not assume that he or she can distinguish between insulin shock and diabetic coma. The general rule is:

Always give sugar; never give insulin.

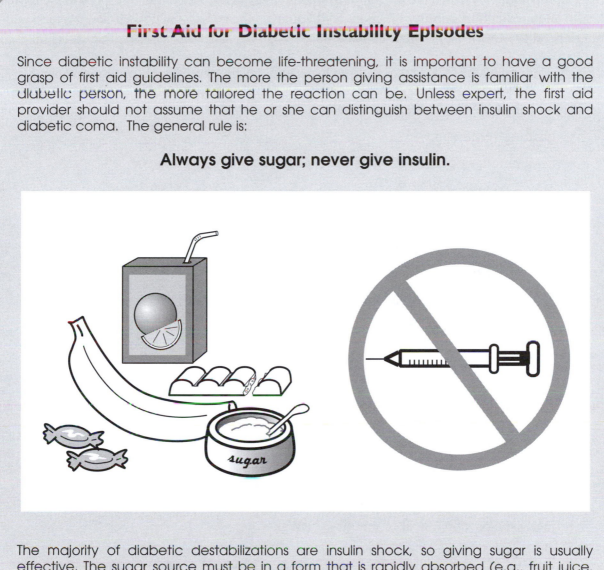

The majority of diabetic destabilizations are insulin shock, so giving sugar is usually effective. The sugar source must be in a form that is rapidly absorbed (e.g., fruit juice, candy/chocolate, banana). If the person is not fully conscious, be cautious about choking risk – place the sweet substance in the cheek pouch or under the tongue.

If it turns out that the person is having a hyperglycemic episode, added sugar will not make a significant difference in the short term. On the other hand, giving insulin if the person is in insulin shock could prove fatal.

Having given sugar, keep the person warm and comfortable and watch for improvement. If you do not see good signs of recovery within 5-10 minutes medical intervention should be sought.

It is important to remember that there is a great deal of individual variation in what leads to hyperglycemic and hypoglycemic episodes. Thresholds can change in the same person based on a number of physical and life circumstances. In general, the better the person's overall health and medication stability the more resilient he or she is, but it is good to be prepared and not depend too much on predictable patterns.

Common examples of factors that can predispose to developing hypoglycemia include:

- incompatible medication type, diabetic medication change
- insulin overdosage
- beginning a new medication of any type (e.g. antibiotic, analgesic)
- drug interactions
- alcohol consumption
- skipping meals/fasting/anorexia
- excessive exercise workouts
- insufficient sleep/sleep disorder/insomnia
- increased stress and anxiety
- significant recent injury

Factors that can predispose to developing hyperglycemia include:

- insufficiently powerful insulin, oral medication dosage is too small
- skipping a dose, irregular medication habits
- drug interactions
- increased psychological or emotional stress
- infection or disease
- alcohol consumption
- high sugar, fast food diet
- thiazide diuretic use
- long-term use of corticosteroid medications
- undiagnosed/untreated diabetes

Quick Guide to Case History Taking for Diabetics

Diabetics can range from having very good health to being quite ill and frail. Case history taking is key to being able to establish a safe and appropriate treatment plan. Very unstable diabetics are not good candidates for massage – it is important to evaluate stability of the diabetic condition and the medication use.

Questions

1. General health, presence of any other conditions.

2. Type of diabetes and date of diagnosis.

3. Progression of the condition. Is it stabilized? Regular medical monitoring?

4. Pharmaceuticals used: insulin, oral medications? Get specifics about types. Taking medications for any other reason? Get specifics.

   Stability of Medication Regimen: Any medication problems? Any recent changes?

   If taking insulin, by injection, pump, or other device? Where are the usual sites? Most recent site?

5. Any recent diabetic crisis? Date, nature of the episode, outcome. Frequency of destabilizations? Best sugar source to use if client destabilizes – does he or she keep a supply on hand? Where? Discuss how to proceed if a destabilization occurs.

6. Kidney and cardiovascular health. These systems are generally compromised in diabetics, especially those who have had the disease for more than 10 years.

   CV System: Hypertension, atherosclerosis, history of heart attack or stroke, heart failure status? Typical BP reading? When last taken and value?
   Kidneys: Frequent kidney infections or stones? Kidney failure status?

7. Peripheral tissue status. Any neurovascular changes: tingling, numbness, reduced sensation anywhere? Leg cramps, muscle weakness? Open sores or lesions – how managed? Any problems with delayed healing? Any history of gangrene? If yes, get details. Any amputations?

8. Any problems with vision? Any other diabetic complications?

9. Any current 'bugs' or infections?

10. Usual home hydro and exercise practices – any MD restrictions on these? Medically supervised exercise plan? Glucose stability usually good during exercise?

11. When was the last dose of medication or insulin taken? Last meal? Last glucose level check? Determine peak stability period.

12. Had massage therapy before? If yes, well tolerated?

Observations

1. Observe for:
   - texture and moisture of the skin
   - areas of discoloration, open sores or lesions
   - fungal infections
   - bruising; inquire about how long it takes to resolve
   - distal edema

2. Check for locations of altered sensation.

3. With advanced cases of diabetes and significant vascular compromise, a 'line of demarcation' may be observed. This is a defined area on the skin, especially on the lower extremity, suggestive of poor tissue distal to the line.

Quick Guide to General Treatment Issues with Diabetic Clients

Treating the client with diabetes for stress reduction or musculoskeletal complaints occurs quite commonly in massage therapy practice. Some general guidelines are offered here. It is important to also take note of the medications related guidelines coming next in this chapter.

1. Therapists must consider the pathophysiologic changes in the vasculature and connective tissues that occur with diabetes mellitus. It is important to have a clear picture of how resilient the tissues are, especially in the extremities, and whether there is sensory loss. Healing times can be prolonged and healing quality may be poor. In the advanced stages of diabetes the connective tissues can be very fragile and easily injured.

2. With a new client shorter specific sessions are recommended at the beginning. This approach gives both therapist and client the opportunity to monitor responses to treatment and make adjustments progressively. Approach hydrotherapy modality use in a similar way.

3. Diabetics are more susceptible to infection and have more difficulty resolving infections. Hygienic practices are a priority, especially around areas of skin fragility or open lesions. Avoid treating vulnerable diabetic clients if you are sick yourself.

4. Keep in mind that there is an increased likelihood of cardiovascular and kidney systems compromise with longerstanding cases of diabetes. Treatment planning needs to take into account the whole picture of the client's health status.

5. Assess the client's stability before each session. Clients will try to be on time for their appointments and sometimes rush to do so. This can precipitate a period of mild hypoglycemia in a diabetic. If a client arrives in a rush, allow him or her to rest for a few minutes and have a light snack or juice as needed to restabilize. Consider whether the treatment plan must be modified for this session or whether it is better to re-schedule the appointment. Diabetic clients should always feel confident that they can reschedule with you rather than receive massage when they are not feeling stable.

Massage Guidelines – Clients Using Medications for Diabetes Mellitus

General Guidelines

1.   Diabetic stability and medication stability are inextricably linked in most diabetics. For treatment planning, hydrotherapy, and exercise recommendation, the key issues revolve around stability, and whether the proposed treatment might promote instability in some way. Consider carefully the general health status of the client, the medications routine, whether there have been any recent medication problems or changes of any type, whether any destabilizing factors are present in the situation (see the information provided earlier in this chapter), and the daily life practices and tolerances of the client.

2. Diabetic clients know when they are experiencing signs of destabilization and are usually able to inform you. Discuss this possible scenario with the client in advance and determine a plan of action. The client should not take medication when destabilizing unless having been specifically instructed to do so by the physician. Any acute destabilization is an absolute contraindication to massage.

3. As a general rule, massage therapy should be avoided during periods of medication change. This applies to changes in medication type, scheduling, or dosage. It is best to monitor the reaction to the new drug therapy for a week or two before resuming massage treatments. Wait until the situation has stabilized, especially with type 1 diabetics.

4. Scheduling of massage treatments must relate well to the type(s) of medication used. Massage, hydrotherapy, and exercise are all stimuli that increase metabolic activity and consequently have the potential to precipitate a hypoglycemic effect. Unless the client has prior experience with massage therapy, it is at first something of a 'guess' how strong the effect might be. Best practice is to determine the peak bioavailability time of the client's diabetic medication and schedule massage appointments then. It is also important for the client to have eaten sufficiently before each session. Discuss these logistics together, and if necessary with the physician, to determine how best to schedule appointments.

5. Diabetics develop cardiovascular and other system complications over time. These often involve medication controls, for example for high blood pressure or heart failure. Keeping in mind that multiple medication mixes will tend to promote a higher incidence of adverse or toxic reactions, be alert for signs and symptoms.

Guidelines Related to Insulin Sites

1. For clients using insulin injections or external pump devices, review the section entitled **Working Around Injection Sites, Skin Patches and Implant Devices** in Chapter 5.

2. Do not apply local hydrotherapy modalities or use any direct manual techniques over recent sites. The various types of insulin have specific onsets of action; massaging or applying hydrotherapy at the site can alter the insulin pharmacokinetics.

3. Insulin dependent diabetics, especially those who have had the condition for some time, often have old injection sites that they have stopped using because of degenerative tissue changes at the site. These tissues tend to be very fibrous on palpation, often have a 'hollowed out' appearance, and lack normal tissue color and temperature. They also generally have poor local sensation. These sites can cause the same types of problems as matted scars do, for example, reducing range of motion, causing painful 'tugging' on nearby structures, and creating pockets of distal edema. The massage therapist may consider using aggressive modalities like deep heat and friction therapy to address such formations. While hydrotherapy, stretching, and direct

manual techniques can play a role in making these tissues more compliant, this type of treatment approach must always be considered carefully in light of the problems with tissue and circulatory integrity that diabetics can have, especially in the extremities. Each case requires cautious thought and consultation as needed.

Guidelines Related to Oral Hypoglycemic Use

1. Sulfonylureas

These drugs can promote more rapid hypoglycemic destabilization. Be on the alert for signs of hypoglycemia, such as tingling in the fingers, headaches, blurred vision, and increased perspiration.

Drug Interaction Alert

Therapists should be aware of the potentially life-threatening drug interaction between the sulfonylurea drugs and members of the NSAID group including aspirin. A type 2 diabetic client with a musculoskeletal complaint may inadvertently use an OTC pain preparation without knowledge of this fact. The NSAIDs and the sulfonylurea drugs compete for the same sites on the plasma protein albumin.[1] With greater binding of the NSAIDs to albumin, more of the sulphonylurea drug remains 'free' or unbonded in the blood. Since the free drug will interact with pancreatic cells to promote insulin release, the client is at risk of developing hypoglycemia (insulin shock).

NOTE: Garlic also seems to increase the levels of insulin in the blood.

Rashes and other skin sensitivity reactions can occur with the sulfonylurea drugs. Do not massage on-site; adapt client positioning to avoid traumatizing the affected skin or increasing discomfort.

Paresthesias can be a side effect of these drugs, resulting in altered sensation and reduced accuracy of client feedback.

2. Biguanides

Generalized fatigue and weakness can be side effects of this group of drugs. You may need to shorten your treatment time or consider more specific regional approaches.

Complaints of muscle cramps, muscle weakness, and numbness and tingling may be related to electrolyte loss or vitamin B12 deficiency. Muscles and their tendons may be hyper-or hypo-responsive to the application of standard manual techniques.

The biguanides are often associated with easy bruising. Technique depths should be modified as a matter of course. Use of more aggressive techniques like muscle stripping, skin rolling, and cross fiber frictions is not advised.

3. **Starch Inhibitors**

Encourage clients to "use the bathroom" before the massage session. Gas and bloating are among the common side effects of these drugs. Therapists must show sensitivity to unexpected episodes of flatulence since this is a side effect of the medication that can be heightened by massage work.

4. **Thiazolidinediones**

Be alert to complaints of fatigue. This group of drugs can cause low blood hemoglobin levels and anemia. When this type of blood disorder is present it is also important to keep in mind that the client will be predisposed to bruising easily.

Headaches and edema are also fairly common side effects of these drugs. If such complaints are not being improved after a reasonable number of massage treatments, recommend medical evaluation.

Hydrotherapy Guidelines

Stability is again the key issue. Consider the client's diabetic stability each time before using a hydrotherapy modality. Begin with mild approaches and proceed carefully.

With advanced diabetic conditions full body systemic hydrotherapy treatments such as whirlpools, saunas, and full baths are not recommended. The heat associated with these treatments increases the workload of the heart and the metabolic demands of the body. Hypoglycemic reactions are likely to occur despite medication controls. Such modalities are also likely to be unsafe based on the cardiovascular status/medications of the client (see Chapter 7).

Remember to identify injection sites and areas of sensory impairment and adjust the hydrotherapy approach accordingly.

Exercise Recommendation

Regular mild to moderate exercise activity promotes glucose utilization by the musculature (decreases blood glucose levels), improves the health of the circulatory system, and builds muscle and bone mass. However, because of the additional glucose uptake by exercising tissues, exercise has the potential to be destabilizing. Types of medication, dosage, and medication routine are important considerations in determining the nature and scheduling of exercise programs. Ask about current activity levels and build the exercise plan around the client's lifestyle. With advanced cases of diabetes it is best to consult with a health care team that provides the services of a qualified exercise therapist.

The sulfonylurea drugs increase skin sensitivity to sunlight, so suggesting protective clothing and exercising in shaded areas will be beneficial.

Gastrointestinal irritations like diarrhea and vomiting can predispose the client to dehydration and electrolyte deficiencies. Encourage proper hydration and nutrient replacement. If muscle cramps or spasms occur the client should stop the activity instead of trying to 'work through it.'

The client may feel generally fatigued and weak. When exercise intensifies these effects, reassess the frequency, intensity, and duration of the exercise program.

1. Freeman Clarke, J.B., et al., *Pharmacological Basis of Nursing Practice*, 4th ed., pg, 810, Mosby Year Book Inc., Missouri, 1993

CHAPTER 9
Drugs for Managing Respiratory Inflammation and Congestion

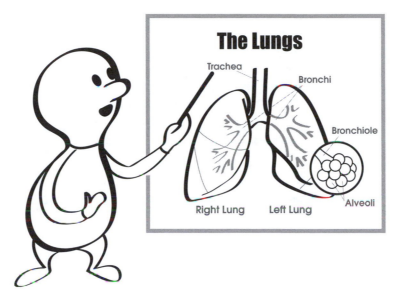

The respiratory system is responsible for the exchange of oxygen and carbon dioxide between the body's tissues and the air. Oxygen is inhaled and added to the circulating blood, while carbon dioxide is removed from the blood and exhaled as a waste product. Any respiratory system factors that disrupt this normal exchange mechanism, such as infection, disease, or chronic irritation, can eventually lead to a form of chronic obstructive pulmonary disease.

Chronic obstructive pulmonary disease (COPD) is a degenerative state involving significant loss of lung competence to perform the function of ventilation. Respiratory conditions that commonly contribute to COPD include asthma, bronchitis, and emphysema. The American Lung Association provides the following statistics, current to 1998, from national surveys and reports about these three conditions:[1,2,3]

- the annual economic cost of asthma is about $12.7 billion dollars
- 14.6 million people report having asthma
- asthma is the most common chronic disease in children and causes about 300 childhood deaths each year
- 8.9 million Americans currently have a physician's diagnosis of chronic bronchitis
- 3 million Americans are diagnosed with emphysema

CONDITIONS THAT COMMONLY CAUSE COPD

Asthma

Asthma is characterized by smooth muscle spasm, inflammation, and increased mucus production in the bronchioles. These are the results of mast cell breakdown to liberate proinflammatory substances including prostaglandins, leukotrienes, bradykinins, and histamine. The overall effect is congestion, compromise of air passage diameters, and impaired respiration. Asthma has both acute (asthma attack) and chronic presentations, and at its most serious can be life-threatening. Shortness of breath, wheezing, and coughing are experienced in varying degrees of severity.

Asthma is usually activated by allergic or hypersensitivity responses to inhaled substances like pollen, pollutants, and dust, but can also be a reaction to ingested foods and some drugs (e.g., aspirin and other NSAIDs, beta blockers), and a sequela of respiratory tract infections. The causes of asthma are not fully understood.

Emphysema

Emphysema is a degenerative condition characterized by the development of large empty spaces (bullae) in place of alveolar clusters, destruction of alveolar capillary beds, and decreased elastic recoil of the lungs. These changes occur over time in response to irritation and damage, mostly from smoking, but sometimes from occupational or other exposures to polluted environments.

Emphysema is a dyspneic condition, meaning that it is characterized by shortness of breath. If the person has a cough it is usually because of concurrent chronic bronchitis in a long-term smoker or presence of an infection. Individuals with emphysema have trouble getting enough oxygen through the lungs and into their body tissues; as the condition progresses they often need supplementary oxygen. The dyspnea is especially noticed when exhaling – the person has to recruit the accessory muscles of expiration.

Chronic Bronchitis

Chronic bronchitis is characterized by increased mucus activity and congestion, productive cough (material is coughed up), and a tendency to recurrent respiratory tract infections. It is a set of degenerative changes in the immune and clearance functions of the bronchial passageways rather than a distinct disease state. Chronic bronchitis is generally diagnosed when, in the absence of other pathologies, a cough is present for at least three months of the year over two consecutive years.

The cause of chronic bronchitis is usually long-term smoking; it can also result from prolonged respiratory irritation/allergies or repeated bouts of acute bronchitis.

Normal respiratory function involves a combination of good gaseous exchange capacity and efficient musculoskeletal action to move the thorax. Respiratory disorders often result in unbalanced use of muscles and stress on joints of the ribcage and thoracic spine, causing muscle and joint discomforts that can bring a client to massage therapy. For example, long-term tightness and overuse of the muscles of inspiration often produces 'barrel chest,' where the thorax is held in an upward, distended position.

Muscles of Inspiration	Muscles of Expiration
Primary diaphragm internal intercostals **Secondary** scalenes sternocleidomastoid pectoralis muscles upper trapezius levator scapula quadratus lumborum	**Primary** none (passive process) **Secondary** abdominals external intercostals low back muscles

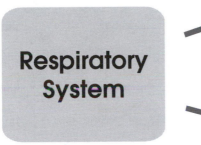

Respiratory System

→ **Upper Respiratory Tract**
consists of nasal cavities, sinuses, pharynx, tonsils, and larynx

→ **Lower Respiratory Tract**
consists of trachea, bronchi, bronchioles, and alveoli

Signs and symptoms of respiratory irritation and disease can include: rhinorrhea (runny nose), face pain and pressure from sinusitis, the sore throat of laryngitis, productive and non-productive cough, chest pain, dyspnea (shortness of breath), increased phlegm and mucus production, musculoskeletal disorders of the neck and thorax, altered breathing patterns, wheezing, reduced tissue integrity and cyanosis in the extremities, and clubbing of the fingertips and nailbeds.

When pharmaceuticals are used to manage respiratory congestion and inflammation the overall effect is to improve clearance of the air passages and optimize conditions for gaseous exchange in the lungs.

The medications discussed in this chapter include those that:

- treat/manage allergic reactions

- increase airway diameter

- manage respiratory congestion

- suppress coughing

1. DRUGS THAT TREAT/MANAGE ALLERGIC REACTIONS

Antihistamines

The antihistamines are used to control the actions of histamine, which is one of the primary mediators of the inflammatory response. Rather than reversing current symptoms, they act to reduce histamine's ability to produce further effects. Many types of antihistamines can be purchased without a prescription, and are sold either alone or in combination with other drugs. Common examples include diphenhydramine (Benadryl) and chlorpheniramine (Chlo-Tripolon).

Histamine

Histamine is an endogenous compound produced and stored in cells, especially mast cells and blood-borne basophils. It is found in most tissues of the body but is especially prevalent in the gastrointestinal tract, in the respiratory and cardiovascular systems, and in certain areas of the central nervous system. Mast cells reside in the connective tissue membranes that surround blood vessels, nerves, lymphatic tissues, and all organs. Other cells that make histamine are found in and around parts of the CNS, in tissues undergoing healing, in the gastric mucosa (mucous membrane), and in epidermal cells.

In order to produce its effects, histamine must be released from the cells that are storing it. Most typically, this happens in response to tissue injury or infection and in allergic (antigen-antibody) reactions. Histamine release usually occurs in the presence of bacteria, viruses, and perceived antigens such as dust, pollen, and some foods, but any number of substances may act as antigens, including pharmaceuticals. Other factors that can cause histamine release include cold, physical exercise, and deep pressure into tissues.

Common reactions to histamine release include runny nose, watery eyes, and itchy skin. The table below lists other more serious effects of histamine.

Body Tissues	Effects of Histamine
Heart	Increases the rate and force of contraction, decreases the atrioventricular conduction rate.
Blood Vessels	Constricts venules, dilates arterioles. This causes plasma leakage and edema formation. Generalized release can lead to hypotension.
Bronchioles	Very powerful bronchoconstrictor. Can cause breathing difficulty.
Exocrine Glands	Increases salivary, bronchial, and lacrimal gland secretion. Also increases nasal mucosa production and secretion.
Gastrointestinal	Increases smooth muscle contraction and gastric secretion; can cause epigastric distress.
Skin	Eczema, purpura, urticaria.
Central Nervous System	Seems to act as a neurotransmitter to generate wakefulness, but its exact role is unclear.

Uses

The antihistamines are used in the management of:

- allergic/hypersensitivity reactions
- motion sickness, nausea, vertigo
- insomnia
- cough
- Parkinsonism and related symptoms

Mechanism of Action

Histamine binds with two cellular receptor sites: H1 and H2 receptors. H1 receptors are primarily located in the gastrointestinal tract, the CNS, and vascular and respiratory smooth muscle, while H2 receptors are largely found in the GI tract and are mainly involved in gastric acid secretion.

Antihistamine drugs compete with histamine for these receptor sites on cell membranes. The antihistamines discussed in this chapter target H1 receptor sites.

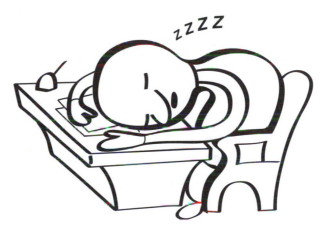

Because histamines cross the blood-brain barrier and occupy receptor sites that seem to be important in wakefulness, drowsiness is a well-known side effect of antihistamine medications. They are sometimes used intentionally to produce sedation. Newer antihistamines such as Hismanal, Claritin, and Seldane have been designed to have less of a sedative effect.

Certain antihistamines (e.g., diphenhydramine) directly suppress the cough reflex center in the medulla. They also seem to affect other CNS receptors, such as those that respond to serotonin and acetylcholine, hence their potential for use in managing some CNS disorders.

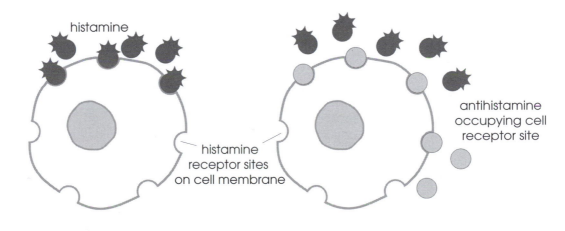

Cromolyn Sodium

Cromolyn sodium stabilizes the membranes of the mast cells in the respiratory tract to prevent release of proinflammatory substances including histamine. It is primarily used to prevent bronchospasm when exposure to allergens or to other known predisposing factors is anticipated. It is utilized alone or in combination with other medications, usually as part of the management of asthma. Cromolyn is administered via a metered aerosol inhaler or by using a spinhaler, which is a small hand-held propulsion device designed to facilitate deep inhalation of medication in powder form.

Commonly prescribed forms of cromolyn sodium include Intal, Intal Inhaler, Nasalcrom, Crolom, and Opticom.

2. DRUGS THAT INCREASE AIRWAY DIAMETER

The diameters of airway passages can be compromised by:

- **inflammation:** Respiratory inflammation is usually caused by allergic/hypersensitivity reactions that result in release of inflammatory mediators such as histamine, thromboxane, and the leukotrienes.

- **hyper-responsiveness of the air passages:** The exact reason for this is unclear, but breakdown of endothelial cells due to irritants like smoking and infections seems to be a contributing factor. Normally these cells produce substances that act as bronchodilators to maintain the size of airway passages. Loss of these cells appears to render the bronchiolar smooth muscle more likely to hyperreact and go into spasm.

- **reflex bronchoconstriction:** Bronchoconstriction typically occurs in the presence of irritating airborne substances, possibly via a protective neural response. In some instances this response appears to become hyper-reactive and the air passages go into excessive constriction.

Drugs used to enlarge airway passages include the:

- bronchodilators
- anticholinergic drugs

Uses

Both drug types can be used to:

- manage asthma, emphysema, bronchitis, bronchiectasis, and other chronic obstructive pulmonary disorders
- manage/prevent exercise-induced asthma
- control allergic/anaphylactic type reactions
- relieve nasal/sinus congestion

Mechanism of Action

- **bronchodilators**

The commonly prescribed bronchodilators fall into two categories:

- the beta-adrenergic agonists or sympathomimetic agents; examples include albuterol (Ventolin), fenoterol hydrobromide (Berotec), and epinephrine HCl (Primatene Mist Solution)

- the xanthine derivatives of which theophylline is the prototype; examples include Theo-24, Slo-bid, Slo-Phylline, and oxtriphylline (Choldeyl)

Beta-Adrenergic Agonists

In Chapter 7 the role of alpha and beta receptors in the cardiovascular system was discussed, and mention was made of similar receptors in the lungs. The lungs have beta-2 receptors on the smooth muscle cells of the respiratory passages. Sympathetic nervous system stimulation of these receptors initiates a complex series of intracellular responses that results in bronchodilation.

Beta-adrenergic agonists mimic the actions of the sympathetic neurotransmitter norepinephrine by stimulating beta-2 receptors to produce dilation of bronchial passages. These drugs also seem to stimulate the respiratory centers in the brain, and to stabilize the membranes of cells like mast cells.

The most effective form of administration of the beta-adrenergic agonists is by inhalation. They are useful during any stage of asthma, and as a pretreatment before exercise or allergen exposure.

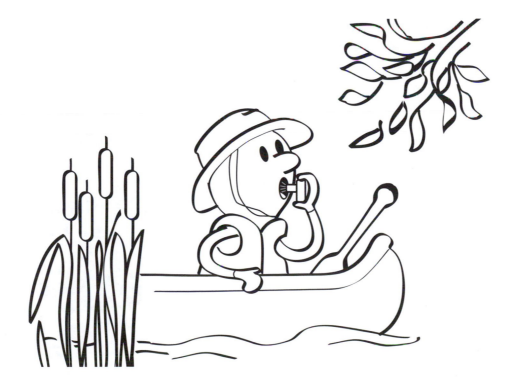

Xanthine Derivatives

The xanthine derivatives, which resemble caffeine in chemical structure, stimulate bronchodilation and improve mucociliary transport function. In addition, they seem to inhibit intracellular activity that leads to smooth muscle cell contraction. Theophylline, the prototype of the group, is also believed to suppress intracellular calcium release and inhibit prostaglandin formation. In combination, these actions improve the size of airway passages and the overall function of the respiratory system.

Mucociliary Transport System (Mucociliary Elevator)

The membranes that line the respiratory passages contain specialized cells whose purpose is to clear foreign particles upward toward the throat. There are two types of cells involved in this function:

- **goblet cells:** produce mucus that entraps the particles
- **ciliated cells:** have hair-like structures called cilia that mobilize the mucus out of the respiratory system

Both types of cells can be damaged or eliminated by chronic irritation. When this happens the person has to rely more heavily on coughing to eject foreign particles.

- **anticholinergic drugs**

In addition to beta-2 receptors, cholinergic receptors are also present in the smooth muscle of the bronchial tree. They react to the neurotransmitter acetylcholine (ACh). When produced by the parasympathetic nervous system, ACh acts on these cholinergic receptors to cause bronchoconstriction. Drugs such as ipratropium bromide (Atrovent) block these sites and reduce bronchoconstriction episodes.

Only a small percentage of respiratory patients (those who do not respond to or who show sensitivity to the beta-adrenergic agonists and xanthine derivatives) use the anticholinergic drugs.

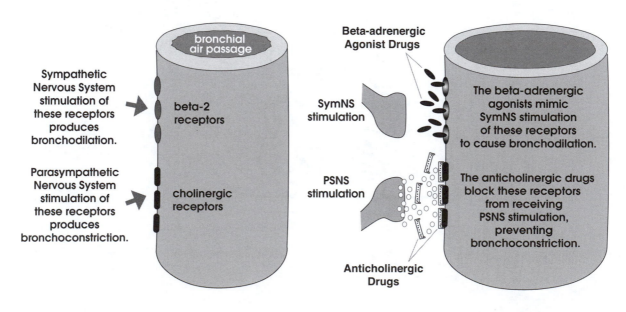

Massage Therapy & Medications

3.   DRUGS THAT MANAGE RESPIRATORY CONGESTION

Congestion of the respiratory passageways due to inflammation, irritation, or infection present (singly or in combination) is typical of many respiratory disorders. Congestion and inflammation of air passages not only reduces their diameter but can also progress to cause poor gaseous exchange in the alveoli.

Signs and symptoms of respiratory congestion include runny nose, increased mucus and abnormal sputum production, and productive cough. The drugs used to manage respiratory congestion and inflammation include:

- decongestants
- expectorants
- corticosteroids

Decongestants

Decongestants act on the blood vessels that supply the mucosa lining the respiratory tract. They stimulate alpha-1 adrenergic receptors located in the blood vessel walls to cause vasoconstriction. Hyperemia, edema, and mucus production are all reduced. These effects increase the size of bronchial and nasal airways and reduce the congestion associated with respiratory disorders.

Decongestants are available in nose drops or nasal sprays, and in oral forms as tablets, capsules, and syrups. Examples of commonly used drugs in this group include oxymetazoline (Afrin, Coricidin), and pseudoephedrine (Sudafed).

Expectorants

Thickened mucus and static mucus plugs can seriously congest the respiratory tract and impair gaseous exchange. Most expectorants (guaifenesin is the most widely used) activate a series of reflexes that stimulate goblet cells in the mucosa to increase fluid production. Other types, such as potassium iodide, act directly on the mucosal cells to produce the same effect. The result is increased mucous flow that loosens accumulated secretions and reduces their viscosity. At the same time the respiratory tract is lubricated. These effects allow the client to produce a more productive and less frequent cough.

Corticosteroids

The corticosteroids control inflammation and have a number of uses in respiratory disease. The availability of these drugs in several forms (aerosol sprays, tablets, injections, etc.) offers versatility in the long-term management of respiratory disorders. The corticosteroids have already been discussed in Chapter 6, and since they pose some concerns for massage treatment planning the reader is advised to review this earlier information.

Bronchitis and bronchial asthma are often managed with corticosteroid nasal sprays. The doses needed in nasal corticosteroids are much smaller than the oral or parenteral ones. It is presently still unclear whether long-term use of these nasal preparations will have the same side effects as oral doses, or lead to hyper- or hyposensitivity of the airways.

4. DRUGS THAT SUPPRESS COUGHING

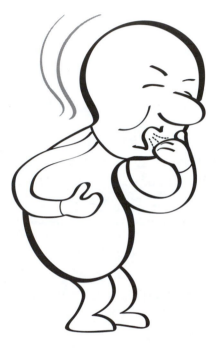

Coughing is a response to irritation of the respiratory tract. It can be either physiologic or voluntary. It aids in removing mucus and irritants to keep the lungs and bronchial tree free of obstructions. A cough should be deep, explosive, and effective in clearing the airways. When problematic coughing episodes disturb sleep or cause pain, cough suppressants, called antitussive medications, are prescribed.

Antitussives

Antitussives prevent or relieve coughing through a variety of means. Some, such as dextromethorpham hydrobromide (DM in cough and cold preparations) and the narcotic analgesics, depress the cough center in the CNS. Others, for example the antihistamine diphenhydramine, inhibit the irritant effect of histamine on the respiratory mucosa, while benzonatate (Tessalon) has a local anaesthetic affect on the respiratory tract.

Decongestants, expectorants, antihistamines, and analgesics are the usual primary ingredients in most OTC cough and cold preparations. In combination they relieve symptoms such as runny eyes and nose, sinus pressure, coughing episodes, and minor musculoskeletal aches and pains.

SIDE EFFECTS – Drugs for Respiratory Disorders

This table lists the common side effects of the groups of medications discussed in this chapter. Therapists must keep in mind that other side effects may occur, and that reactions will vary in degree and intensity. Always ask clients about incidence and intensity of any side effects experienced. When more than one medication is being taken, whether in the same drug group or not, therapists should appreciate the increased potential for adverse and idiosyncratic effects.

Side Effects	AH	BD	CS	AT	DC	EX
Abdominal Cramps						XX
Allergic Reactions				X		
Altered Taste		XX			X	
Anemia	XX					
Angioedema		XX	XXX			
Anorexia	XX				X	X
Anxiety	X	XX			X	
Appetite Changes		X			X	
Blurred Vision	X					
Blood Dyscrasias	XX			X		
Bradycardia		XX			XXX	
Breathing Difficulty	X	XXX	XXX		XXX	
Bronchospasm		XXX	XXX			
Bruising		XX				
Chest Pains		XXX			X	
Chills	XX					
Cold Extremities		XX				
Confusion	X					
Constipation	XX					
Cough		X	X			
Drowsiness	XX		X			
Dry/Sore Eyes	X		X	X		
Dry Nose	X				X	
Dry Mouth/Throat	X	X	X	X	X	
Diarrhea	X					X
Dizziness	XX	XX	XXX	X	X	X
Dysrhythmia		XX				
Dysuria					X	
Facial Flushing						XX
Fatigue	XX		XX	X		
Fever	X	XX	X	X		XXX
GI Bleeding or Pain				X		
Hallucinations		XXX			XXX	

Side Effects	AH	BD	CS	AT	DC	EX
Headaches	XX	XX	XXX		X	X
Hypertension		XX			X	
Hypotension		XX				
Insomnia	XX	X				
Irregular Heartbeat		XX			X	
Joint Pain			XXX			
Lightheadedness	X	XX			X	
Liver Dysfunction				X		
Mood Changes		XX				
Muscle Cramps		XX				
Muscle Weakness	X		XXX			
Nausea	XX	XX	XXX			X
Nasal Stinging					XX	
Nasal Stuffiness	XX		X		X	
Neuritis	XX		X			
Numbness		XX				
Palpitations					XX	
Paresthesia	XX					
Photosensitivity	XX					
Rashes	XX		XXX			X
Restlessness	X	X			X	
Seizures		XXX			XXX	
Shortness of Breath		XXX	XXX		XXX	
Sore Throat			X			
Sweating	XX	X			X	
Tachycardia		XX			X	
Thrombocytopenia	XX					
Tinnitus	XX					
Tremors	X	XX			X	
Urinary Freq. Changes	XX		XXX		X	
Vomiting	X	X	X		X	X
Weakness					X	
Wheezing	XX	XX	XX			

AH: Antihistamines, BD: Bronchodilators, CS: Cromolyn Sodium, AT: Antitussives, DC: Decongestants, EX: Expectorants

X – tolerable – notify medical practitioner if bothersome
XX – serious – monitor closely and notify medical practitioner
XXX – very serious – seek medical attention

Quick Guide to Respiratory System Case History Taking

Compromise of the respiratory system results in reduced availability of oxygen and poor removal of carbon dioxide, both of which can adversely affect the health of all the tissues and systems of the body. It is especially important to note that diminished oxygen delivery to body cells and resistance to blood entering the lungs place greatly increased stress on the heart. Congestive heart failure is a common co-finding in long-term respiratory disorders.

Questions

1. Identify the respiratory disorder(s) for which the client is being treated. Time frame since diagnosis? Progression of the condition?

2. How is the condition managed? Generally well stabilized? Medications, herbal remedies, lifestyle changes, exercise regimen, etc.

3. If asthma or allergies, is it clear what the triggers/antigens are? Be thorough in asking about allergies or sensitivities to oils, aromas, or other elements present in your clinic environment.

4. Have there been any recent crises or hospitalizations? If yes, get details. Discuss how to proceed if such an occurrence were to take place.

5. Is a pharmaceutical delivery device like an inhaler being utilized? Does the client need to keep it handy during treatments? How is it used?

6. Other means of pharmaceutical delivery, e.g., skin patch?

7. Health of other body systems? Ask in particular about the heart (see Quick Guide in Chapter 7) and blood pressure. Any other systemic disorders? How managed? Medications for other disorders? Any drug combining issues?

8. Regular medical monitoring? When was the last physician visit?

9. Activity and energy levels? Exercise tolerance? Breathlessness episodes?

10. Have any restrictions been placed on exercise or hydrotherapy?

11. Smoking and drinking habits? (These can be aggravating factors.)

12. Sleep habits? Apnea? Any positions that are not comfortable to lie in?

13. Does stress have an impact on the condition?

14. Tissue health, especially in the extremities? Is healing time slower for cuts or injuries? Any numbness or sensory impairment?

15. Aches and pains related to the condition? Postural problems?

Observations

1. Observe thoracic posture for hyperkyphosis, barrel chest, pigeon chest. Is there spinal immobility, head forward posture?

2. Status of the muscles of respiration and spinal and thoracic joints - do the muscles look tight or prominent? Does the person move stiffly? Is breathing visible, effortful?

3. Breathing patterns – apical, diaphragmatic, shallow, rapid? Mouth or nose breather? Listen for wheezing sounds, watch for shortness of breath.

4. Observe for coughing, runny eyes, nose, etc.

5. Tissue health – look for bruises, varicosities, edema, etc. Skin and nail beds – pallor, cyanosis, and fingernail clubbing are signs of hypoxia.

Quick Guide to Working with Clients with Compromised Respiratory Systems

Treating clients with respiratory complaints is not uncommon for the massage therapist. Massage can be helpful in addressing musculoskeletal concerns, in promoting relaxation, and sometimes in reducing congestion. Keep drinking water and Kleenex handy.

- Massage is not appropriate during an acute episode like an asthma attack, or if there is an infection with fever.

- Consider the client's cardiovascular status and adapt massage and hydrotherapy approaches accordingly. The combination of a chronic respiratory disorder and a weakened heart can 'double up' on causes of dyspnea, high blood pressure, fatigue, and so on. *hunger for breath*

- Consider the integrity of the body tissues. With any long-term respiratory disorder the tissues will tend to be more fragile and more easily injured; when injured they will heal more slowly and with a poorer quality of repair.

- Shorter treatments are suggested at first to give both therapist and client an opportunity to monitor responses to therapy. If unsure about how best to design a treatment plan given the person's health status, consult with the physician.

Client Positioning

- Nasal stuffiness, sinusitis, and other types of upper respiratory congestion are most compatible with semi-supine or seated positions.

- Asthmatics may have difficulty lying flat in either prone or supine position because of a feeling of not being able to get enough breath.

- Sidelying position is useful for treating the intercostals and abdominal oblique muscles and is sometimes a preferred position for asthmatics.

- Towel rolls/small bolsters can be used to stretch thoracic structures during massage treatment. Place a comfortably sized 'roll' widthwise across the table so that when the client lies back onto it the positioning will be just below the inferior angles of the scapulae (head level should not be lower than the sternum). If the client finds this position too uncomfortable, adjust the roll to a smaller size or try a rolled towel laid lengthwise under the spine.

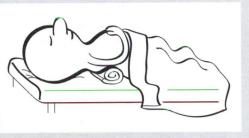

Choice of Techniques

- Clients will generally benefit from specific work to the muscles of respiration and the joints of the thoracic spine. Direct manual techniques may need to be modified if there is significant tissue fragility. Used appropriately, rib springing and joint play can also be highly effective in mobilizing stiff joints.

- Tapotement on the back can reflexly trigger coughing episodes; it also appears to promote bronchospasm, so it is not a good technique to employ with asthmatics. Clients with lower respiratory tract congestion, for example from bronchitis or emphysema, can benefit from the use of heavy tapotement to promote clearance, although intense coughing may be triggered. This work is generally done in prone position with a large number of pillows under the body and torso (the head is tilted somewhat downward) to promote drainage. This specialized technique is usually performed by physical therapists – massage practitioners must refer clients out for this work or consult carefully before proceeding. Note that both the position and the technique are not appropriate if there is significant cardiovascular disease.

- Drainage techniques, including specialized lymphatic drainage if the therapist has been trained, can be very useful in treating sinusitis or other types of upper respiratory congestion.

Muscle strains, nerve impingement syndromes, and rib fractures and dislocations can severely restrict respiratory function. In many instances the client will benefit from massage therapy. It is important to keep in mind that such clients are often taking anti-inflammatories, cough suppressants, analgesics, and possibly other types of medications to manage pain and inflammation.

Massage Guidelines – Clients Taking Medications for Respiratory Disorders

General Guidelines

1. Keep in mind that clients with respiratory disorders are often taking pharmaceuticals in addition to respiratory medications, especially if they have cardiovascular problems. Also, preparations geared to respiratory complaints may contain a number of drugs that can influence massage treatment planning.

2. NSAID medications can intensify asthma. A client may use an OTC aspirin or ibuprofen product for a musculoskeletal complaint, experience more breathing difficulty, and as a result increase asthma medication use. Such situations should be referred to the physician for further evaluation.

3. Side effects of dizziness, lightheadedness, and postural hypotension are common to most of the medications discussed in this chapter. Monitor the client and be prepared to shorten the treatment. Give specific post-treatment instructions to move slowly and carefully when sitting up and getting off the massage table.

4. The drugs discussed in this chapter all have the potential to create or add to breathing difficulties like shortness of breath, wheezing, and bronchospasm. Position the client comfortably and allocate more time to work on the muscles of respiration. If the client complains that breathing difficulty is increasingly becoming a problem, suggest medical follow-up.

5. Dryness of the respiratory passages and mouth can cause episodes of throat irritation and coughing during treatments. Keep some drinking water handy.

Specific Guidelines

1. Antihistamines

Central nervous system depression can compromise the normal responses of connective tissues to manual techniques that involve deep pressure and stretching. Inquire about the degree of drowsiness or fatigue present from the antihistamine use – this information is your guide to determine the degree of CNS depression. If the client is experiencing considerable fatigue or sleepiness you will probably need to give shorter treatments with a more stimulating rather than relaxing focus.

Paresthesias, neuritis, and muscle weakness may occur. These require the practitioner to modify depth of technique. Keep in mind that client feedback might be misleading. Hypersensitive tissue areas should not be treated locally until the sensitivity has decreased.

If anemia is present as a side effect of antihistamine use the client may bruise more easily.

2. **Cromolyn Sodium**

Angioedema reactions and skin rashes may be symptoms of a systemic allergic response to this drug. The affected tissues become edematous and painful. Depending on the intensity of the reaction the massage appointment may need to be rescheduled until the situation is stabilized. If massage treatment is possible, ensure that the client is positioned comfortably and avoid direct contact with the sensitive areas. Keep in mind that nearby tissues may also be tender to pressure.

Client complaints of joint pain and muscle weakness may be related to side effects of this drug. Assess/consult to determine if such complaints are actually drug side effects.

Changes in urinary function often occur. The client may need to interrupt the treatment to use the washroom.

3. **Bronchodilators**

Cardiovascular and respiratory problems such as blood pressure changes, chest pain, irregular heart beat, wheezing, and bronchospasm need to be monitored carefully. If the doctor has evaluated these side effects and the client is okay for massage, adapt the treatment to avoid causing additional stresses. Do not use tapotement, especially on the back, since it can trigger exaggerated cardiovascular and respiratory reactions.

Numbness and vascular changes like increased bleeding time can occur with bronchodilator use. Observe for signs of bruising and modify depth of technique.

Occasionally bronchodilator medications cause seizure disorders. Determine how the situation is being managed and ensure that massage therapy is appropriate. If yes, schedule your treatments to maximize medical stability.

4. **Decongestants**

Elevated heart rate and changes in blood pressure are the main concerns with decongestant use. Stay informed about any cardiovascular system reactions the client may be having and take blood pressure routinely. Review the guidelines in Chapter 7.

Seizures are also an occasional complication of decongestant use.

5. **Antitussives and Expectorants**

Dextromethorpham can cause altered sensory perception. The client may not give accurate feedback about technique depth or hydrotherapy temperatures, and may be prone to episodes of lightheadedness and disorientation. When such symptoms are present to a significant degree, massage treatment can be an additional stress on the body. Postpone massaging until after the physician has evaluated the medication use.

Since corticosteroids and narcotic analgesics can be utilized for their decongestant and antitussive effects, refer to the information in Chapter 6 about these drugs. Their use can have a number of implications for massage treatment design.

Hydrotherapy Guidelines

Before treating clients with respiratory conditions, make sure you are aware of any medically indicated hydrotherapy restrictions. These may be related to a number of factors, including cardiovascular status, medications being used, and asthma sensitivities.

Identify any sensitivities to essential oils and bath additives before beginning hydrotherapy treatments. If unsure, start with water modalities only and introduce additives gradually. Keep in mind that people with breathing difficulties may find the more intense hydrotherapy modalities overwhelming.

If the client has medication-induced hypotension, systemic heat treatments are not appropriate. This issue is discussed in more detail in Chapter 5.

Decongestant medications raise a concern about the use of heat treatments like steams and saunas. Normal heat dissipation responses to temperature can be compromised, and the heart may react in an erratic manner (palpitations, dysrhythmias, rising blood pressure). Monitor blood pressure during any hydrotherapy modalities used.

Decongestant nose drops and sprays have more localized effects, but these should also be taken into account in hydrotherapy decision-making. For example, facial steams can be very effective in relieving upper respiratory tract congestion, but when a local decongestant is being used, blood vessels in the nasal passages will not vasodilate normally in response to the heat stimulus.

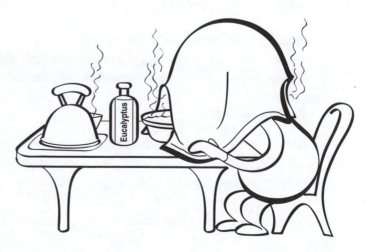

Cough suppressant medications like dextromethorpham and codeine can alter temperature perception. All hydrotherapy treatments should be modified and the client should be carefully monitored throughout the treatment.

Mustard poultices are often used on the chest to reduce respiratory tract congestion, especially with chronic bronchitis.

Exercise Recommendation

Several of the drugs prescribed for respiratory conditions can cause side effects like muscle cramps and joint pain. Exercise can intensify these complaints without the client or practitioner making the connection to a medication side effect. It is important to be aware of the profiles of the drugs being taken before recommending exercises.

Antihistamines and decongestants can increase perspiration during exercise. Confirm that the client understands the need to drink enough fluids and avoid becoming overheated.

Cardiovascular and respiratory problems like heart palpitations, hypertension, shortness of breath, and bronchospasm can be worsened by exercise. Determine what the client's normal activity levels are and plan a program that is compatible.

Exercise prescription for the seriously compromised respiratory patient is a specialized field. When a client has advanced emphysema, bronchitis, or asthma it is best to work with a health care team that provides the services of a qualified exercise therapist.

1. American Lung Association, *Trends in Asthma Morbidity and Mortality,* January 2001 www.lungusa.org/data/asthma/asthmach_1.html#economic

2. United States Environmental Protection Agency, *Asthma and Upper Respiratory Illness* www.epa.gov/children/asthma.htm

3. American Lung Association, "Estimated Prevalence of Lung Disease," *Lung Association Report April 2001*   www.lungusa.org/data/lae_01/lae.html#bronchitis

CHAPTER 10
Drugs for Managing Mood and Emotional Disorders

The Canadian Mental Health Association describes mental illness as "the single largest category of disease affecting Canadians." According to a study published in Chronic Diseases in Canada[1] in 1998, depression and distress cost Canadians at least $14.4 billion per year in treatment, medication, lost productivity, and premature death.

Mood and emotional disorders are also referred to as **affective disorders**, which are sub-categorized into several distinct medical conditions. For the purposes of this text the focus will be on anxiety, depression, and psychosis.

Everyone experiences episodes of anxiety and depression that arise from life situations, for example:

- before a major exam
- having to give a speech to one's peers
- following the death of a loved one
- after losing a job

These bouts of altered mood are usually normal and short-lived. They are part of change and personal growth processes. During such times medications are sometimes used on a short-term basis. However, when mood disturbances have a serious affect on health and well-being, psychotherapy and ongoing medication treatment may become necessary.

Research suggests that biochemical imbalances in the brain contribute to disturbances of mood and emotion. Chiefly involved are the neurotransmitters, which are molecules produced in and released from nerve cells (neurons). They cross the synaptic gaps between neurons in order to transmit signals from cell to cell. When these transmitters are available as needed and in balance with each other, they play an important role in normal expression and stabilization of emotion. Alterations in the actions, influence, and availability of several neurotransmitters have been associated with specific mood disorders. The neurotransmitters most commonly involved appear to be gamma-aminobutyric acid (GABA), serotonin, norepinephrine, and dopamine.

NEUROTRANSMITTERS COMMONLY IMPLICATED IN MOOD AND EMOTIONAL DISORDERS

Gamma-Aminobutyric Acid (GABA)

GABA is present in all parts of the CNS. There are two types of receptors for GABA: GABA-A and GABA-B. Stimulation of the A type of receptor causes an increase in intracellular chloride ion concentration; when the B receptors are stimulated cell membrane permeability to potassium is altered. GABA's effects are inhibitory – it is considered the CNS's primary inhibitory neurotransmitter. Anti-anxiety drugs such as the benzodiazepines mimic the inhibitory actions of GABA through acting on the A receptors.

Serotonin (5-hydroxytryptamine or 5 HT)

Serotonin is found in three major body areas: in blood vessels, in the intestinal wall, and in the central nervous system. Within the CNS, serotonin functions as an inhibitory neurotransmitter and is involved in the regulation of mood, appetite, body temperature, sleep, and sexual function. It also plays a role in pain control and suppression. Fourteen main sub-types of serotonergic receptors have being identified. Reduced serotonin levels have been correlated with aggressive behavior, irritability, sleep disorders, depression, and eating disorders. Antidepressant drugs such as Prozac enhance serotonin functions.

Dopamine

Dopamine, synthesized in various areas of the CNS including the hypothalamus, the basal ganglia (primarily in the substantia nigra), the frontal lobes, and the limbic system, influences mood by producing the pleasurable sensations that accompany behaviors like sex, eating, and being in control. It increases secretion of the hormones corticotropin and growth hormone and inhibits the release of prolactin. Many chronic diseases result from overproduction or underproduction of dopamine. Parkinson's Disease, for example, is a condition of dopamine underproduction. Symptoms of schizophrenia can occur when dopamine flow throughout the nervous system is compromised. There are at least five types of dopamine receptors. Several pharmaceuticals are used to improve dopamine function in the CNS, including the anti-psychotic drug Thorazine.

Norepinephrine

Norepinephrine is also known as noradrenaline. It is a neurotransmitter found in the autonomic nervous system (ANS) and generally in the CNS. A portion of the body's norepinephrine supply is produced from dopamine and released from areas located in the pons and medulla of the brainstem. The supply for the ANS is largely manufactured in the adrenal medulla. There are about eleven subtypes of norepinephrine receptors. Depending on the type of receptor being stimulated, norepinephrine can have inhibitory or excitatory effects. It is believed to play a role in regulation of several functions including mood, arousal, focus, alertness, and blood pressure control. It may be responsible for some symptoms of depression.

synapse

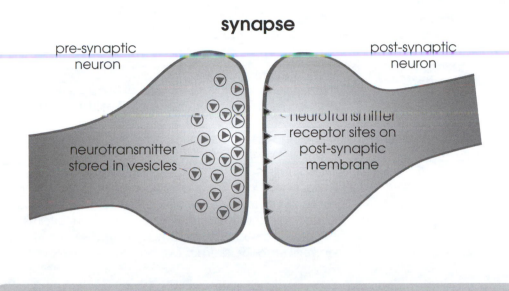

pre-synaptic neuron

post-synaptic neuron

neurotransmitter stored in vesicles

neurotransmitter receptor sites on post-synaptic membrane

Each neuron produces its own neurotransmitter, which it stores in specialized vesicles. Stimulation of the pre-synaptic neuron results in the neurotransmitter substance being released into the synapse. It traverses the 'gap' to the post-synaptic neuron where it occupies its receptor sites. Depending on whether the transmitter is an inhibitory or excitatory chemical, the post-synaptic neuron is either inhibited or excited. Once the neurotransmitter has relayed its message it is removed from the synapse.

The drugs used to treat anxiety, depression, and psychosis produce their therapeutic effects by targeting neurons, their receptors, and neurotransmitter activity in a variety of ways. Medications used to manage mood and emotional disorders fall into three main categories:

- anxiolytic or anti-anxiety agents

- antidepressants

- antipsychotic drugs

1.   THE ANTI-ANXIETY MEDICATIONS

Results of a 1999 study sponsored by the Anxiety Disorders Association of America showed that the total cost of anxiety disorders in the United States, including misdiagnosis and undertreatment, is more than $42 billion a year.[2] More than 19 million Americans suffer from one or more anxiety disorders, making them the most common of all mental illnesses. According to the National Institute of Mental Health,[3] there are several classifications of anxiety. The table on the next page outlines the general signs and symptoms of each.

Anxiety Disorder Classification		Characteristics
Panic Disorder		Episodes of intense fear that strike often and without warning. Physical symptoms include chest pain, heart palpitations, shortness of breath, dizziness, abdominal distress, feelings of unreality, and fear of dying.
Obsessive-Compulsive Disorder		Repeated unwanted thoughts or compulsive behaviors that seem impossible to stop or control.
Post-Traumatic Stress Disorder		Persistent symptoms that occur after a traumatic event such as a rape or other criminal assault, war, child abuse, a natural disaster, or a crash. Symptoms include nightmares, flashbacks, numbing of emotions, depression, anger, irritability, distraction, and being easily startled.
PHOBIAS	Specific Phobia	Experience of extreme, disabling, and irrational fear of something that poses little or no actual danger.
	Social Phobia	An overwhelming and disabling fear of scrutiny, embarrassment, or humiliation in social situations.
Generalized Anxiety Disorder		Constant and exaggerated worrisome thoughts and tension about routine life events and activities, lasting at least six months. The person tends to anticipate the worst even though there is little reason to expect it. Physical symptoms include fatigue, trembling, muscle tension, headache, and nausea.

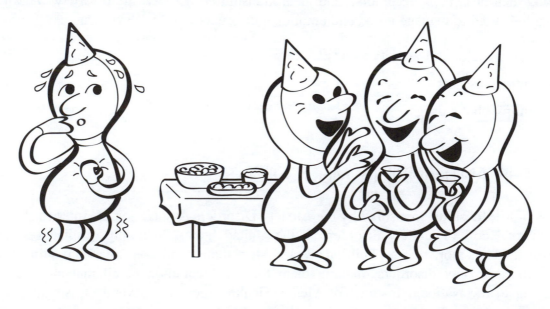

Clients complaining of anxiety related symptoms such as tension headaches, backache, insomnia, and fatigue often use a combination of medications and massage therapy to help control their anxiety.

The medications most commonly used to reduce anxiety include:

- the benzodiazepines
- buspirone HCl (BuSpar)

> In the past, drugs such as the barbiturates and chloral hydrate were used extensively in the management of mood disorders, including anxiety. The barbiturates can produce serious side effects like respiratory depression and cardiovascular shock, while chloral hydrate creates dependency with long-term use. These drugs are now largely replaced by the much safer benzodiazepines for mood disorder treatment. The barbiturates are presently used in the management of various forms of epilepsy and as an adjunct to general anaesthesia.

Benzodiazpines

Commonly prescribed drugs in this category include: diazepam (Valium), lorazepam (Ativan), alprazolam (Xanax), and ketazolam (Loftran).

Uses

The benzodiazepines are used in the management of:

- short-term anxiety related conditions
- insomnia
- tension headaches
- stress related muscle tension, spasms, and pain
- various medical disorders characterized by seizures or convulsions

Mechanism of Action

The benzodiazepines depress all areas of the central nervous system to produce effects ranging from muscle relaxation and mild sedation to deep sleep. In very large doses coma and even death can result.

The precise mechanism of action of these drugs is not completely understood, but they appear to enhance the inhibitory actions of GABA. When GABA binds to its receptor sites on the neuron membrane it initiates a series of reactions to increase chloride ion influx into the cell. Higher intracellular chloride concentration causes neurons to become hyperpolarized, meaning that they are more difficult to activate. GABA is believed to act in this manner on both pre- and post-synaptic neurons in all areas of the brain to depress CNS discharge levels. The benzodiazepines stimulate GABA receptors to produce the same effect.

Buspirone HCl

Buspirone HCl (BuSpar) is different chemically and pharmacologically from the benzodiazepines. It reportedly has fewer CNS side effects, does not exert anticonvulsant, sedative, or muscle relaxant effects, and has less abuse potential than the benzodiazepine group.

Uses

Buspirone HCl is indicated for:

- generalized anxiety disorders
- short-term relief of anxiety related symptoms

Mechanism of Action

Buspirone is a relatively new drug whose mechanism of action is not known. It does not affect GABA receptors but instead appears to have:

- a high affinity for serotonin (5-HT1A) receptors
- a moderate affinity for brain dopamine receptors

Its anti-anxiety effects begin to be felt after about two weeks.

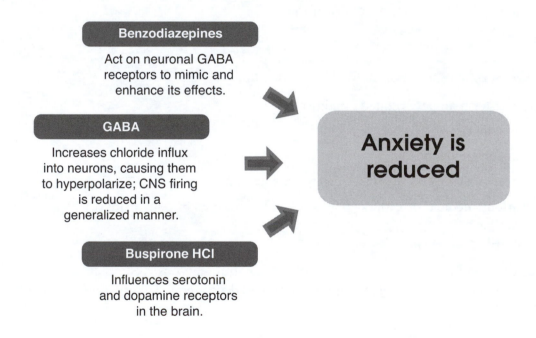

2.   THE ANTIDEPRESSANTS

The World Health Organization (WHO) estimates that by the year 2020 depression will be the number two cause, second only to ischemic heart disease, of "lost years of healthy life" worldwide. It is currently estimated that 340 million people suffer from depression globally, of whom 17-20 million are in the U.S. population.[4]

Studies indicate that the cost of clinical depression exceeds $47.3 billion annually in the United States. One out of every five adults will experience a depression episode at some time, and women are twice as likely as men to suffer from bouts of depression. Everyone including children can be affected.[5]

GENERAL SIGNS AND SYMPTOMS OF DEPRESSION

Persistent sad mood

Loss of interest in ordinary activities

Loss of interest in sex

Decreased energy, fatigue

Sleep disturbances

Eating disturbances (loss of appetite and weight, or weight gain)

Difficulty concentrating and remembering

Poor self confidence

Difficulty making decisions

Feelings of guilt, worthlessness, helplessness

Thoughts of death and/or suicide

Suicide attempts

Irritability

Excessive crying

Chronic aches and pains that do not respond to treatment

Decreased productivity

Absenteeism

Alcohol and drug abuse

Type of Depression	Characteristics
Major Depression (clinical depression)	Most common type of depression. At least five of the major symptoms of depression are present.
Dysthymia	Second most common type of depression. A milder form – sufferers may present with only two or three symptoms and are often undiagnosed and undertreated. Can last two years or more.
Bipolar Depression	The depressive phase of a manic-depressive mood disorder, in which the person experiences extreme highs and lows. Symptoms are very similar to major depression.
Seasonal Affective Disorder	Usually occurs in the winter months and is associated with absence of sunlight. Tends to resolve in the spring and summer months. Typical symptoms include loss of energy, decreased activity, sadness, and excessive eating and sleeping.
Other	Post-partum, drug induced, pain induced, endogenous, and reactive types.

More information about the types of depression can be obtained through the Internet or local mental health support groups.

The following groups of medications are used alone or in combination in the management of depression:

- antidepressants
- anti-anxiety medications (see previous section)
- lithium carbonate
- antipsychotic drugs (discussed in the next section)

The commonly prescribed antidepressants include:

- the tricyclic antidepressants
- the selective serotonin re-uptake inhibitors (SSRIs)

The Tricyclic Antidepressants

The most common drugs in this group are: amitriptyline (Elavil), imipramine (Tofranil), and doxepin (Sinequan).

Uses

The tricyclic antidepressants are used in the management of:

- depression
- anxiety related conditions
- various compulsive or obsessive disorders
- migraines and chronic muscle tension headaches
- sources of neurogenic pain, such as cancer pain and peripheral neuropathy
- attention disorders, hyperactivity, and enuresis (bed wetting) in children 6+
- other conditions: peptic ulcers, narcolepsy, bulimia nervosa, cocaine withdrawal

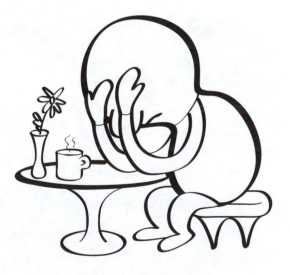

Mechanism of Action

The biochemical model of depression in use until recently suggested that concentrations of serotonin and norepinephrine were low and therefore post-synaptic neuroreceptors were not being sufficiently activated. The current belief is that post-synaptic neurons seem to create more serotonin and norepinephrine receptors, making them supersensitive to these molecules. It is this supersensitivity that leads to the symptoms of depression.

The tricyclic antidepressants produce their effects by inhibiting re-uptake of norepinephrine and serotonin molecules that have been released into synapses. This increases the volume of these transmitters in the synaptic gaps. With more neurotransmitter substance in their synapses post-synaptic neurons are even further stimulated. This super-stimulation causes their membranes to 'down-regulate.' Restoration of normal sensitivity of post-synaptic neurons improves the quality of signals traveling among the different parts of the brain, and balances and normalizes the reactions of the neuroreceptors to their neurotransmitters.

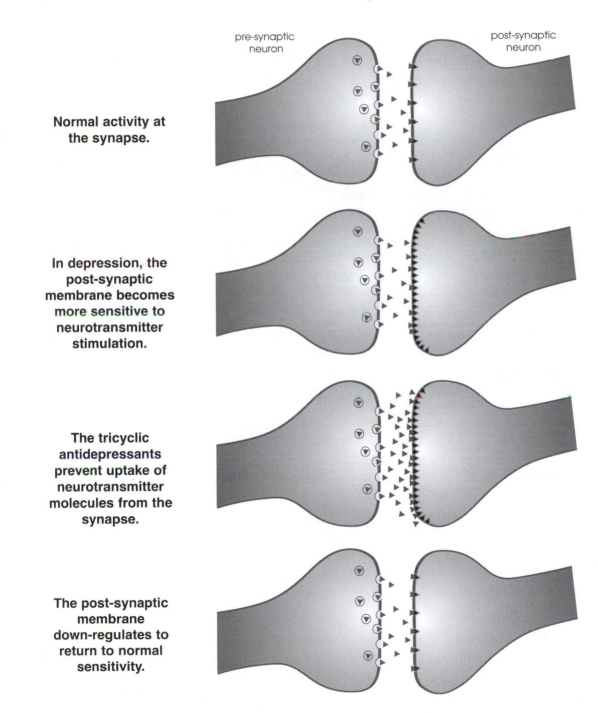

The tricyclic antidepressant mechanism of action

The therapeutic effect of the tricyclic antidepressants, that is reduction of depression symptoms, begins to occur after a minimum of 2-3 weeks. This lag is believed to correspond with the time it takes the post-synaptic neuromembranes to down-regulate.

Serotonin Selective Re-Uptake Inhibitors (SSRIs)

This is a relatively new but already extensively used group of drugs that includes: fluoxetine (Prozac), paroxetine (Paxil), and sertraline (Zoloft).

The SSRI mechanism of action is similar to that of the tricyclic antidepressants except that SSRIs selectively inhibit the re-uptake of serotonin. The effects of these drugs also become apparent 2-3 weeks after the start of therapy. The SSRIs are credited with a safer profile than the tricyclic drugs.

Recent Developments

Two new medications, called venlafaxine (Effexor) and nefazodone (Nefadar, Serzone, Serzonil), have been introduced into the marketplace recently and are being increasingly used in depression management. Although their exact mechanisms of action are still unclear, venlafaxine appears to be a potent re-uptake inhibitor of serotonin and norepinephrine and a weak inhibitor of dopamine re-uptake. Nefazodone displays re-uptake inhibition of both serotonin and norepinephrine but not dopamine. Although the end result is similar to that of the tricyclic antidepressants, these drugs appear to have a safer profile, comparable to the SSRIs.

Lithium Carbonate

Lithium carbonate, manufactured as Carbolith, Duralith, Eskalith, Lithane, and Lithizine, is a more specialized type of antidepressant.

Uses

Lithium is used either alone or in combination with other medications to manage:

- manic depressive (bipolar) depression
- vascular headaches

Mechanism of Action

Lithium is the drug of choice in managing bipolar depressive syndromes, but its actions are not fully understood. Several theories[6] exist regarding its mechanism of action. One suggests that lithium ions accumulate inside neurons by entering via their sodium channels. The cells have difficulty removing them, and increased intracellular lithium concentrations result in decreased neuron excitation. Another theory is that lithium serves as a second messenger to engage processes that reduce the excitability of neurons. It is also suggested that lithium may affect synaptic serotonin concentrations. Whatever the mechanism, lithium helps normalize the production, concentration, and metabolism of serotonin and norepinephrine. The resulting stabilizing effect on the patient occurs in about three weeks.

> ## Lithium Toxicity
>
> Lithium dosage has to be carefully monitored medically because of the close relationship between therapeutic and toxic doses. There are a number of symptoms of lithium toxicity: diarrhea, drowsiness, loss of appetite, muscle weakness, nausea and vomiting, slurred speech, confusion, clumsiness, blurred vision, dizziness, severe trembling, and increased urination.
>
> Lithium is reabsorbed in the kidneys in a manner very similar to sodium. When less sodium is passing through the kidney tubules, such as during heavy sweating, lithium reabsorption will actually increase. This can lead to toxic levels of lithium if sodium is not actively replaced.

3. THE ANTIPSYCHOTIC MEDICATIONS

Psychosis is a major emotional disorder characterized by personality disintegration and loss of contact with reality.[7,8] The cause is somewhat unclear, although several contributing factors have been identified. These include genetic inheritance, environmental factors, CNS biochemical imbalances, viral infections, and social predisposition. Most researchers believe that psychotic behavior is related to an imbalance of the neurotransmitter dopamine.

Schizophrenia is the most common type of mental illness involving psychotic behavior. Some of the symptoms of schizophrenia include delusions, hallucinations, unusual movement patterns, and disorganized thinking and actions. The 1996 total cost of treating schizophrenia in the United States, including direct treatment and societal and family costs, was about $65 billion. Schizophrenia affects one percent of the population, consumes a fourth of all mental health costs, and accounts for one in three psychiatric hospital bed occupancies.[9]

> ## Dopamine Theory of Psychosis
>
> The dopamine theory of psychosis postulates that too much dopamine is being produced in the limbic system and in other areas of the CNS. This excess dopamine is absorbed by the post-synaptic neurons, and the symptoms of schizophrenia result for reasons that are not entirely clear. The role of antipsychotic medication is to prevent excess dopamine from entering these neurons.

Types of Schizophrenia	Characteristics
Paranoid	Preoccupation with one or more delusions or frequent auditory hallucinations Feelings of persecution
Negative or Deficit	Lack of initiative, motivation, social interest, enjoyment, emotional responsiveness

Catatonic
(must have at least two symptoms)
	Immobility, stupor
	Excessive motor activity
	Extreme negativism
	Mutism
	Peculiarities of voluntary movement
	  (voluntary assumption of inappropriate or bizarre postures)
	Stereotyped movements
	Prominent mannerisms, grimacing
	Echolalia
	  (compulsive repetition of words spoken by someone else)
	Echopraxia
	  (compulsive imitation of the actions of others)

Residual	Grossly disorganized or catatonic behavior Absence of prominent delusions, hallucinations, disorganized speech
Disorganized	Disorganized behavior, disorganized speech, flat affect Disturbance in behavior, communication, and thought Lack of any consistent theme Unusual mannerisms and facial expressions

This section will focus on two categories of drugs used to manage psychosis:

- the typical antipsychotic drugs
- the atypical antipsychotic drugs

Antipsychotics are often used in combination with other CNS medications, for example anti-anxiety drugs or lithium.

Typical Antipsychotic Drugs

This drug group is known as the phenothiazines. They are among the oldest antipsychotic medications and are still widely used today. The most commonly prescribed include: chloropromazine (Largactil, Thorazine), haloperidol (Haldol), and trifluoperazine (Stelazine).

Uses

The phenothiazines are used in the management of:

- psychotic disorders, for example schizophrenia, or for patients with explosive or hyper-excitable behavior
- short-term management of severe psychotic depression with anxiety
- elderly patients with multiple symptoms such as anxiety, agitation, tension, fears, depressed mood, and sleep disturbances
- severe nausea and vomiting
- intractable hiccups

Mechanism of Action

These drugs act at all levels of the central nervous system to interfere with the effects of dopamine. They occupy and block dopamine receptor sites on post-synaptic neurons. Their effects include altering responses to dopamine in parts of the brain like the mesolimbic area, which is important to emotions and mood.

Two main effects are achieved with the phenothiazines:

- a tranquilizing effect that occurs soon after the drug is administered, characterized by profound quiet and calm
- an anti-psychotic effect that takes 2-3 weeks to develop, characterized by normalization of thought, mood, and behavior

The sedative, anti-anxiety, and antiemetic (control of vomiting) properties of the phenothiazines are related to their global inhibitory impact on the CNS, including on the reticular activating system and the chemoreceptor trigger zone.

HYDROTHERAPY ALERT

The phenothiazines suppress the hypothalamic centers that regulate central and peripheral temperatures. Regulation of both hot and cold are affected. In hot and humid conditions the sweating mechanism is compromised and the person can develop heat stroke. In cold environments, hypothermia can develop.[7] These effects pose serious concerns related to the use of hydrotherapy, as will be discussed later in the chapter.

Atypical Antipsychotic Drugs

In 1989, clozapine (Clozaril) became the first of this group of drugs to receive FDA approval as an antipsychotic medication. Subsequently, risperidone (Risperdal), olanzapine (Zyprexa), and sertindole (Serlect) have also come onto the market.

Mechanism of Action

The antipsychotic effects of these drugs seem to be produced more selectively at specific CNS locations. For example, clozapine acts on dopamine receptors in the limbic areas of the brain. Risperidone and olanzapine influence specific dopamine and serotonin sites. The actions and effects of the atypical antipsychotic drugs give them a generally safer drug profile than the traditional phenothiazines.

SIDE EFFECTS – Drugs for Mood and Emotional Disorders

This table lists the common side effects of the groups of medications discussed in this chapter. Therapists must keep in mind that other side effects may occur, and that reactions will vary in degree and intensity. Always ask clients about incidence and intensity of any side effects experienced. When more than one medication is being taken, whether in the same drug group or not, therapists should appreciate the increased potential for adverse and idiosyncratic effects.

BZD: Benzodiapines, BUS: Buspirone, TCAD: Tricyclic Antidepressants, LI: Lithium, PHZ: Phenothiazines, SSRI: Selective Serotonin Reuptake Inhibitors, ATAP: Atypical Antipsychotic

Side Effects	BZD	BUS	TCAD	LI	PHZ	SSRI	ATAP
Abdominal Cramps			X	X			
Acne				X		XX	
Agranulocytosis							XXX
Allergic Reactions	XXX						
Alopecia		X				XX	
Akathisia*					XXX		
Angina						XX	
Anorexia	X		X				
Anxiety	X		X			XX	
Asthma						XX	
Ataxia	XX			X	X		
Appetite Changes	X		XX			XX	
Arthritis						XX	X
Blood Dyscrasias	XXX				XXX		XXX
Blurred Vision	XX	X	XXX		XXX	XX	XX
Bone Pain						XX	
Bradycardia			XXX	XXX		XX	
Breast Pain					XX	X	
Breathing Difficulty		XX		XXX			XX
Bronchitis						XX	
Bursitis						X	X
Cardiac Arrest					XXX		
Cramps		X					X
Chest Pains & Congestion		XX					
Chills						X	X
Cough						X	
Cold Extremities				XXX		XX	
Confusion	XXX	X	XXX	XXX	X		
Constipation	XX	X	XXX			X	
Convulsions				XXX		XXX	
Decreased Sweating					XXX		
Depression	XXX	X					
Dreams –Vivid						XX	
Diarrhea	XX	X	X	XXX		XX	
Dizziness	XX	X	XX		X	XX	
Drowsiness	XX		XX	XXX	X	XX	
Dry/Sore Eyes			XX		X		XX

Side Effects	BZD	BUS	TCAD	LI	PHZ	SSRI	ATAP
Dry Mouth	X	X	XX	X	X	XX	
Dry Skin		X					X
Dry Throat						XX	
Dystonia*					XXX		
Dyspnea						X	X
Edema		X		XX		XX	X
Euphoria						XX	
Eye Pain			XXX			X	X
Fatigue	X	X				XX	
Fever	XXX	X				X	X
GI Discomfort		X					XX
Hallucination	XXX					XX	
Headaches	X	X	XX	X	X	X	
Heat Stroke					XXX		
Hepatitis			XXX		XXX		
Hypertension			XXX			XX	
Hypotension	X		XXX	XX	XX	XX	
Increased Appetite			X			XX	
Increased Sweating		X	X			X	
Increased Salivation							X
Insomnia	XX	X	X			XXX	
Irregular Heartbeat		XX	X			XX	X
Joint Pain						XX	
Laryngospasm					XXX		
Libido Changes	X	X	XXX		X	XXX	X
Lightheadedness	XX	XX			XX	X	
Liver Dysfunction+	XXX				XXX		
Memory Impairment	XXX						
Menstrual Pain, Cycle Chgs		X			X	XX	X
Migraine							X
Mood Changes						XX	
Muscle Cramps		X		X	X		X
Muscle Weakness	XXX	XX		XXX	X	XXX	X
Myocardial Infarction		XXX				XX	
Nausea	X	X		XX		X	X
Nasal Stuffiness		X			X		
Neck Pain						X	X
Nervousness						XX	
Nosebleeds						X	X
Numbness		XX				XX	
Palpitations	X		X			XX	X
Paresthesia						XX	
Photosensitivity			X		XX		X
Postural Hypotension	XX		X		X	XX	XXX
Pruritus		X	X			XX	
Pseudoparkinsonism*					XXX		
Psychosis							XX
Pupil Dilation	X		X				
Rashes	XXX	X			X	XX	

Side Effects	BZD	BUS	TCAD	LI	PHZ	SSRI	ATAP
Respiratory Depression					XXX		
Respiratory Infection						X	
Restlessness			XXX			XX	
Sedation	X					XX	XXX
Seizures	XXX				XX		XXX
Slurred Speech				XXX			
Sore Throat	XXX	X					
Stroke		XXX					
Tachycardia	X		XXX	XXX	XXX	XX	
Tardive Dyskinesia*					XXX		X
Taste Changes		X	XX	X		X	X
Thrombocythemia							X
Thrombophlebitis (inj)	X						
Thirst				X			X
Thyroid Function Chgs				XXX			
Tinnitus	X	X	X				X
Tiredness (unusual)	XXX			XXX	XXX	XX	
Tremors	X	X	XXX	XXX		XX	
Uncontrolled Movements	XXX				XXX		
Unusual Bleeding	XXX					XXX	
Urinary Frequency Chgs	XX		XXX	XXX	XX	XX	
Viral Infection						XX	
Vomiting	X		X	XXX		XX	X
Weakness (unusual)	XXX		XX	XXX	XXX	XX	
Weight Gain		X	XX	XXX	X	XX	
Weight Loss						XX	X

BZD: Benzodiapines, BUS: Buspirone, TCAD: Tricyclic Antidepressants, LI: Lithium, PHZ: Phenothiazines, SSRI: Selective Serotonin Reuptake Inhibitors, ATAP: Atypical Antipsychotic

+ **liver dysfunction:** jaundice-like symptoms including yellow eyes and skin

* **akathisia:** restlessness, need to keep moving

dystonia: muscle spasms of the face, neck and back, tic-like or twitching movements, twisting movements of the body, inability to move the eyes, weakness of arms and legs

pseudoparkinsonism: difficulty speaking and swallowing, loss of balance, shuffling walk, mask-like face, stiffness of arms and/or legs, trembling of hands and fingers

tardive dyskinesia: lip smacking or puckering, puffing of cheeks, rapid or worm-like movements of the tongue, uncontrolled chewing movements, uncontrolled arm and leg movements

X – tolerable – notify medical practitioner if bothersome

XX – serious – monitor closely and notify medical practitioner

XXX – very serious – seek medical attention

Quick Guide to Case History Taking

Clients will not always be open about mental health problems they are experiencing. Recognition of medications and symptom presentations can help the practitioner identify areas needing diplomatic exploration. Therapists must be able to define the fine line between obtaining necessary treatment planning data and prying into personal information.

Questions

1. Identify the mood disorder(s) for which the client is being treated.

2. When was the diagnosis made?

3. Is the cause known? Are current life stressors a factor?

4. Clarify the medications being taken. Is the condition well stabilized on these medications?

5. If the client has musculoskeletal complaints, could they be related to the condition or to medication use? Has this been evaluated medically?

6. Inquire about organ system health. For example, the cardiovascular system can be stressed by emotional disorders and by several of the medications used to manage them.

7. Does the client have a good support system?

8. What are the goals of the client in seeking massage treatment?

9. Any past experience with massage therapy? What was the response to it? Any concerns or reservations about receiving massage?

10. Inquire about where the client "holds stress." Try in a diplomatic way to identify sensitive areas that might be difficult for the client to have touched.

11. Inquire about destabilizing factors like lack of sleep, poor diet, work stress, and alcohol consumption.

Observations

1. Is the client cooperative when answering your questions? Can you establish rapport and get the information you need to proceed?

2. How focused or attentive is the client?

3. Pay attention to postural holding patterns. They can give clues about specific areas of tension, past experience of trauma, and overall emotional state.

4. Observe how the client breathes – shallow rapid breathing often signals stress.

5. Inquire about any visible bruises and scars. These may be related or unrelated to the mental health problem; bruises may reflect medication side effects.

Quick Guide to Working with Clients Who Have Mood Disorders

Working with clients with mood disorders can be challenging. It is important to mutually agree on the nature of the therapeutic relationship being entered into and the scope of massage therapy practice as it applies in each case. Ideally, the massage therapist will be only one of a team of health care practitioners the client is seeing. The massage therapist needs to show sensitivity and acceptance, and to maintain good professional boundaries to avoid dependency or issues arising from unrealistic expectations of massage therapy. The guidelines for working with clients with mood disorders are not necessarily different from other scenarios, but additional awareness, sensitivity, and diplomacy are called for.

1. The client must understand the treatment plan and feel informed about the techniques you are going to use and on what body areas. If the client specifically indicates not wanting a part touched, always respect this request. Focus your efforts on developing trust and ease in the therapeutic relationship. When the client is ready to evolve the treatment he or she will let you know.

2. Be a good listener, but do not exceed your scope of practice or your personal comfort zone. Work in concert with the other health care practitioners involved with the client's case.

3. Shorter treatments are suggested for first time clients – this gives everyone an opportunity to monitor the response to therapy. Progress the treatment plan slowly and in frequent communication with the client. Be prepared to stop treatments before the scheduled time if the client is feeling emotionally overwhelmed by the massage work. If unsure about appropriate treatment plan design, consult with the attending physician.

4. Ensure the treatment room is warm and comfortable and external noises are eliminated or reduced to a minimum. Encourage relaxing breathing techniques, beginning with diaphragmatic breathing. Pillow for comfort, keeping any musculoskeletal complaints or medication effects in mind.

5. Show sensitivity to the client's requests or feelings of vulnerability. Be clear that it is the client's decision to disrobe for treatment at his or her level of comfort. You may want to treat in supine position (or other position preferred by the client) until he or she is more at ease with massage. It is important for the client to feel in control of such options.

Choice of Techniques

1. Avoid use of techniques that are deep and aggressive. Such techniques, in addition to the medication-related bruising risk, can jeopardize the client's feeling of safety and cause increased anxiety.

2. The overall effect of your choice of techniques should be nurturing and relaxing. Be especially careful when working on areas you know to be sensitive ones – the techniques used, whether very gentle or more standard, need to have the qualities that feel appropriate to the client.

3. Be mindful of how you handle or hold the client's limbs. Certain manners of treatment or specific positions may trigger negative responses. Always inform the client about what you are going to do.

General Guidelines

1. Check the side effects profile for each drug the client is taking. Toxicity or other adverse reactions are a concern with several of the drugs used to manage mood and emotional disorders. Stay aware of all the medications being taken and be alert for unexpected symptoms or known adverse indicators.

2. Complaints of headaches or muscle and joint pain are typical with most of the drugs discussed in this chapter. If you have been asked to address such complaints but after a few treatments there is no improvement, consult with the medical doctor. You may be trying to treat a side effect.

3. Side effects of dizziness, drowsiness, and lightheadedness in varying degrees of intensity are common to most of the medications used to treat mood disorders. Massage treatment can heighten these symptoms. Be prepared to shorten your treatment time. Give the client specific instructions about getting on and off the table, especially to move slowly after the treatment.

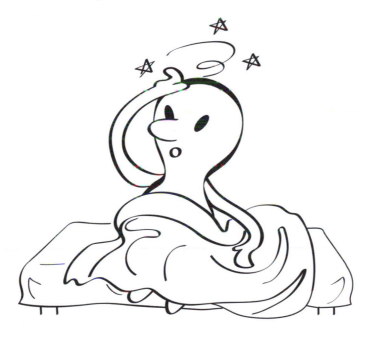

4. Changes in heart rate and blood pressure, and chest pains, strokes, and heart attacks can be related to side effects of several of the mood disorder drugs. Monitor the blood pressure and be alert to changes in skin color, breathing, or pulse that could indicate increasing stress on the heart. When the client is vulnerable cardiovascularly, assess the impact of CV medications being used and avoid treatment approaches that could add to the heart's workload (reference Chapter 7).

5. Mood disorder medications are frequently administered by injection. If your client receives 'shots,' review the appropriate section in Chapter 5.

Specific Guidelines

1. **Benzodiazepines**   *lorazepam*

    Unusual bleeding can occur with these medications. Modify your depth of pressure to avoid causing bruising. Keep in mind that the client may not give accurate feedback about technique depth due to the benzodiazapine CNS depressing effect.

    Exercise caution when stretching muscles and mobilizing joints. Stretch receptor responses will be compromised and the muscles more easily injured. They may also go into reflex spasms more readily.

    Feeling unusually tired or weak can be a side effect of the benzodiazapines. Before treating, inquire about whether the physician has evaluated these symptoms. If not, it is probably better to re-schedule the appointment. If yes, you may need to shorten your treatment time or adjust to a 'lighter' treatment design.

2. **Tricyclic Antidepressants and SSRIs**

    The client may appear restless during the massage. Be prepared for more frequent position changes and perhaps more conversation than is customary.

    Complaints of muscle cramps and spasms can be related to electrolyte loss from diarrhea. In this situation, aggressive manual work or stretching techniques may cause tissue trauma.

    Paresthesias and unusual bleeding can occur with the SSRIs. Modify your depth of pressure and observe for signs of bruising. Client feedback may be misleading.

3. **Phenothiazines**

    Some clients experience muscle spasms, dystonia, and various types of movement incoordination. Working deeply into affected muscles or stretching muscle spasms may not be appropriate. Do not use strong heat applications to relax the tissues since these drugs alter responsiveness to temperature stimuli. Soothing relaxation work is most helpful.

    Laryngospasm and/or tight feelings in the throat and anterior neck can also occur with phenothiazine use. Attempting to 'loosen' the neck directly may cause more anxiety and increase the discomfort.

4. **Atypical Antipsychotics**

    Low blood pressure and orthostatic hypotension are a particular concern with this pharmaceutical group. Give appropriate instructions concerning getting up after the massage session – the client may need assistance.

    There can be complaints of shortness of breath. If the client is comfortable with the idea, spend focused time treating the muscles of respiration.

A side effect of these medications, called agranulocytosis (a drop in the white blood cell count), can result in immune system compromise. The client will likely complain of fatigue and weakness, and will be at increased risk of developing infections. The client might present in a weakened state of health, with the muscles, joints, and other connective tissues feeling more sensitive. Modify your depth of pressure, and be prepared to shorten your treatment. Avoid treating such clients when you yourself are ill.

Some people experience seizures when taking the atypical antipsychotics. If this is the case, determine how the seizure disorder is being managed and whether the client's condition is stable enough for massage. If so, decide on a treatment schedule that is best suited to the medical stability of the client.

5.   Lithium

Be alert for signs or complaints that suggest lithium toxicity. This is a serious concern and presence of such symptoms requires immediate medical evaluation. If you suspect lithium toxicity is occurring, do not massage until the physician gives the 'all clear.'

Hydrotherapy Guidelines

Inquire whether the client has been given any condition or medication related temperature restrictions; ask about daily bath/shower tolerances and if there are areas of sensory impairment. Many of the drugs discussed in this chapter affect the health of the cardiovascular system in some way. Take blood pressure readings before and after hydrotherapy treatments and monitor the client closely during the application. When unsure, discuss the proposed procedure with the physician.

The benzodiazepines depress all areas of the CNS. With CNS depression vascular responses to hydrotherapy modalities can be altered. Using modified temperatures and local versus systemic treatments is recommended.

The tricyclic antidepressants and SSRIs cause increased sweating. This can be a particular concern if the client is also experiencing bouts of diarrhea. Dehydration and low electrolyte levels can result. Modify temperatures and application times and monitor the client closely, making sure he or she is sipping water during the treatment.

Lithium can approach toxic levels under conditions that cause heavy sweating. Systemic hydrotherapy modalities like steams, saunas, hot baths, and sweating herbal wraps are not recommended.[9] Review the signs and symptoms of lithium toxicity presented earlier.

The phenothiazines impair the body's temperature regulating mechanisms. Systemic hot and cold hydrotherapy modalities are contraindicated. Do not use intense heat to relax muscle tension – the client may be unable to give accurate feedback and is at risk for burning at lower than expected temperatures. Local cold applications like cryotherapy can also cause tissue damage.

Exercise Recommendation

A progressive aerobic exercise program can be very helpful in managing the effects of anxiety and depression. Improved circulatory and aerobic capacities aid in increasing energy and appetite, and in improving the quality and quantity of sleep.

Some degree of muscle weakness is a side effect of virtually all the drugs discussed in this chapter, especially the benzodiazepines and lithium. Adjust the intensity, frequency, and duration of the exercises prescribed. Encourage the client not to overexercise.

Low electrolyte levels and dehydration can be a concern with the tricyclic antidepressants and SSRIs. Make sure the client knows the importance of being adequately hydrated and properly nourished for exercise, as well as not becoming overheated.

Vigorous exercise, especially in hot conditions, is not recommended for clients using lithium. Increased sweating and dehydration can lead to lithium toxicity.

When phenothiazine use is producing spasmodic or dystonic symptoms in the client's muscles, it is important to be cautious about recommending strengthening exercises, especially those incorporating weights.

Because the phenothiazines affect temperature control mechanisms in the hypothalamus, vigorous exercise, especially in hot environments, is not recommended. As well, clients taking the phenothiazines must pay particular attention to spending too long in direct sunlight. The metabolites from these medications accumulate in the skin and can react with sunlight to produce a deep blue-black discoloration.

Ensure your client's exercise program has medical approval.

1. Stephens, T. & Joubert, N., "The Economic Burden of Mental Health Problems in Canada," *Chronic Diseases in Canada*, 22(1), Mental Health Promotion Unit of Health Canada, 2001 www.hc-sc.gc.ca/hpb/lcdc/publicat/cdic/cdic221/cd221d_e.html

2. Anxiety Disorders Association of America, "Misdiagnosis of Anxiety Disorders Costs U.S. Billions," 1999 panicdisorder.about.com/gi/dynamic/offsite.htm?site=http://www.adaa.org/dyna/view.cfm%3FID=5

3. National Institute of Mental Health   www.nimh.nih.gov/anxiety/anxiety/idx_fax.htm#top

4. "Depression: A Global, National and Personal Burden" www.depressionresources.ofinterest.com/depression/article.htm

5. National Mental Illness Screening Project   www.nmisp.org/dep/depfaq.htm

6. United States Pharmacopeial Convention Inc., *USP DI, Drug Information for the Health Care Professional*, Volume1B, 12th ed., 1992

7. *Tabers Cyclopedic Medical Dictionary*, 16th ed., F.A. Davis Company, Philadelphia, 1989

8. Freeman Clarke, J.B. et al., *Pharmacologic Basis of Nursing Practice*, 4th ed., Mosby Year Book Inc. Missouri, 1993

9. "U.S. Health Official Puts Schizophrenia Costs at $65 Billion," *The Schizophrenia Homepage* www.schizophrenia.com/news/costs1.html

CHAPTER 11

Drugs for Managing Cancer

The diagnosis of cancer is among the most feared of all diagnoses. Cancer affects everyone's life in some way and places a tremendous burden on society. According to the National Cancer Institute of Canada,[1] there will be an estimated 134,100 new cases and 65,300 cancer deaths in 2001. The most frequently diagnosed cancers are breast cancer for women and prostate cancer for men. The leading cause of cancer death is lung cancer; the most common childhood cancer is leukemia.

In the United States, cancer is second only to cardiovascular disease as a cause of death. Cancer costs for the year 2000, including health care expenditures and lost productivity, are estimated at $107 billion.[2] It is projected that in 2001 over 1.2 million Americans will be diagnosed with cancer and as many as 552,000 will lose their lives to it. The number of new cancer cases is expected to increase by 29% by the year 2010.[3]

Defining Cancer

Cancer is a generic term used to describe over 200[4] malignant diseases whose common characteristic is uncontrolled tissue growth and spread of abnormal cells.

During normal cell life, cells grow, divide, perform their functions, and eventually die. This cycle is directed by genes, hormones, and specific intercellular communications that dictate cell sizes and numbers consistent with their tissue functions. When these controls are disrupted, whether by environmental, genetic, or lifestyle influences, cells can become renegades. Acting outside normal constraints, they begin to multiply rapidly to form new tissue masses called neoplasms or tumors. Tumors can arise from any cell type and are broadly grouped into two categories: benign and malignant.

Benign tumors are not classified as cancer. They do not invade tissues or spread to other body parts. They are usually successfully removed surgically, or if located in a difficult spot, with laser treatment. Malignant, or cancerous, tumors are much more dangerous. Cancer tissues do not respect tissue boundaries. They invade neighboring structures and shed cells that can migrate to distant sites to form new cancers.

Distinguishing Features of Benign and Malignant Neoplasms

Benign	Malignant
Have an expansile growth pattern, enlarging locally within their host structure.	Have an invasive growth pattern, overrunning host stroma and other tissue structures.
Are usually contained within a capsule. Do not spread to distant sites.	Can invade body cavities and blood and lymph channels, leading to spread to secondary sites (metastasis).
Cell turnover is slower.	Cell replication is rapid and frequently abnormal.
Cells are usually fairly well differentiated.	Poor differentiation and maturation of cells is typical, including a tendency to regress to pre-differentiated or ancestor cell types (anaplasia).

Reprinted with permission from Massage Therapy and Cancer, Curties-Overzet Publications Inc., 1999.

Naming Cancerous Neoplasms

Malignancies that originate from epithelial tissues like skin and glandular membranes are referred to as carcinomas, while those associated with mesenchymal tissues such as bone, muscle, and some organs are called sarcomas. Cancers arising from the blood have names ending in the suffix 'emia' as in leukemia, while those that derive from lymph cells are called lymphomas. Cancers are also sometimes named after individuals, for example Kaposi's sarcoma.

Treatment of Cancer

There are many approaches to treating and managing cancer, some of which are contentious or experimental. The current standard medical approach involves:

- surgery
- radiation
- drug therapy

While only one or two of these therapies may be utilized for some cancers, cancer treatment protocols often incorporate a combination of all three.

Surgery is considered the most effective of the three treatments. If the malignancy is operable and diagnosed early enough, surgery can remove all of the cancerous tissue and result in a cure. However, surgery becomes less effective when there are a number of disseminated tumors.

Radiation is the second most effective cancer therapy. Cells that are rapidly dividing are very sensitive to radiation, and cancerous growths contain continually replicating cells.

Radiation therapy is best suited to cancers that are not disseminated and small in size. It is primarily used to 'clean up' any remaining cancer cells after surgery, to shrink tumors to make them more operable, and to control growth of inoperable tumors. Radiation has its dangers and is used in precise locations in controlled doses – sites are often ink-marked or tattooed for exact future reference.

Drug Therapy

While in some cases drug therapy is the treatment of choice, usually pharmaceuticals are employed when the cancer is less amenable to treatment by surgery and radiation, in other words when it has spread. Drugs are also often used when there is a statistical probability that an identified tumor may already have metastasized.

Drug therapy for cancer consists of:

- **Chemotherapy**

Chemotherapy is defined as the use of chemicals/pharmaceuticals to destroy cancerous cells. It is a systemic treatment directed at disseminated cancers.

- **Immunotherapy and Biological Response Modifiers (BRMs)**

This category includes compounds like interferons, interleukins, and other biologic substances that can be used to enhance the individual's immune response. They work best in combination with radiation and chemotherapy.

In the general scheme of cancer treatment management, drug therapies are usually collectively referred to as chemotherapy, and that is how we will refer to them in this text.

Goals of Chemotherapy

Chemotherapy is used with various goals[5] in mind, including:

- achieving a cure
- preventing or controlling cancer spread
- slowing tumor growth
- providing pain relief and otherwise improving quality of life

Depending on the type and location of the cancer, the oncologist selects the chemotherapy approach most likely to be effective. There is a myriad of pharmaceuticals to work with. Some drugs are designed to target rapidly replicating cells to disrupt their reproduction cycle, while others inhibit tumor growth and viability.

For your reference, the table on the next pages, although by no means complete, lists common cancer types and the names of drugs[6] typically used singly or in combination to treat them.

Common Cancer Drugs by Cancer Type

Type of Cancer	Drug
Bladder	Pacis (BCG, live) Valstar (valrubicin)
Brain	Gliadel (carmustine wafer)
Breast	Aredia (pamidronate disodium) injection Arimidex (anastrozole) Aromasin (exemestane) Ellence (epirubicin hydrochloride) Fareston (toremifene citrate) Femara (letrozole) Herceptin (trastuzumab) Nolvadex (tamoxifen citrate) Taxol (paclitaxel) Taxotere (docetaxel) Xeloda (capecitabine)
Colorectal	Camptosar (irinotecan hydrochloride) injection Celebrex (celecoxib)
Head and Neck	Ethyol (amifostine) injection
Kaposi's Sarcoma	Panretin (alitretinoin) gel 0.1% DaunoXome (daunorubicin citrate liposome) Taxol (paclitaxel) injection
Leukemia	Busulfex (busulfan) Campath (alemtuzumab) Daunorubicin HCl (daunorubicin hydrochloride) Gleevec (imatinib mesylate) Neupogen (filgrastim) Mylotarg (gemtuzumab ozogamicin) Trisenox (arsenic trioxide)
Lung	Ethyol (amifostine) Etopophos (etoposide phosphate) Gemzar (gemcitabine HCl) Hycamtin (topotecan hydrochloride) FocalSeal-L Surgical Sealant Photofrin (porfimer sodium) Taxol (paclitaxel) Taxotere (docetaxel)

Massage Therapy & Medications

Type of Cancer	Drug
Lymphoma	Elliotts B Solution (calcium chloride, dextrose, magnesium sulfate, potassium chloride, sodium bicarbonate, sodium chloride, sodium phosphate, dibasic) Intron A (interferon alfa-2a) Rituxan (rituximab) Ontak (denileukin diftitox) Targretin (bexarotene) UVADEX (methoxsalen sterile solution, 20 mcg/ml)
Ovarian	Doxil (doxorubicin HCl liposome) injection Hycamtin (topotecan HCl) Taxol (paclitaxel)
Pancreatic	Gemzar (gemcitabine HCl)
Prostate	Lupron Depot (leuprolide acetate) Nilandron (nilutamide) tablets Novantrone (mitoxantrone hydrochloride) Trelstar Depot (triptorelin pamoate) Viadur (leuprolide acetate implant) Zoladex (goserelin acetate implant)
Miscellaneous Products e.g. for: side effect control immune system strengthening encouraging repair processes	Actiq (fentanyl citrate) – analgesic Anzemet (dolasetron mesylate) – antinausea Blenoxane (bleomycin sulfate) Ceprate SC Stem Cell Concentration System DepoCyt (cytarabine liposome) injection Dostinex (cabergoline) Duraclon (clonidine hydrochloride) Fludeoxyglucose (F-18) injection Isolex 300 and 300i Magnetic Cell Selection System Kytril (granisetron) Levulan Kerastick (aminolevulinic acid HCl) Neumega (oprelvekin) Quadramet (samarium sm 153 edtmp) Sandostatin LAR® Depot (octreotide acetate) injection Temodar (temozolomide) Zofran ODT (odansetron) – antinausea Zometa (zoledronic acid) injection Zyloprim (allopurinol sodium)

The Cell Cycle

Before delving more deeply into the mechanisms of action of the anticancer drugs, an overview of the cell cycle is needed.

With the exception of the permanent cells (muscle and nerve), all cells proliferate by moving through the **cell cycle**. Stable cells, which make up most body structures, only reproduce when new cells are needed. Labile cells, constituting for example the skin, hair, and membranes lining systems like the gastrointestinal tract, reproduce constantly.

The cell cycle is divided into several phases: G1, S, G2, M, and G0. Each phase is characterized according to the intracellular activity that occurs. The G phases are growth, normal activity, and rest phases. With the enzyme RNA polymerase influencing DNA structure, several important proteins and enzymes are produced. The G phases also serve as check-in points for the cell, when the viability of newly created cellular elements is evaluated to see if any repairs or corrections are necessary. During the S phase DNA is replicated, and in the M phase the cell undergoes division to form two identical daughter cells.

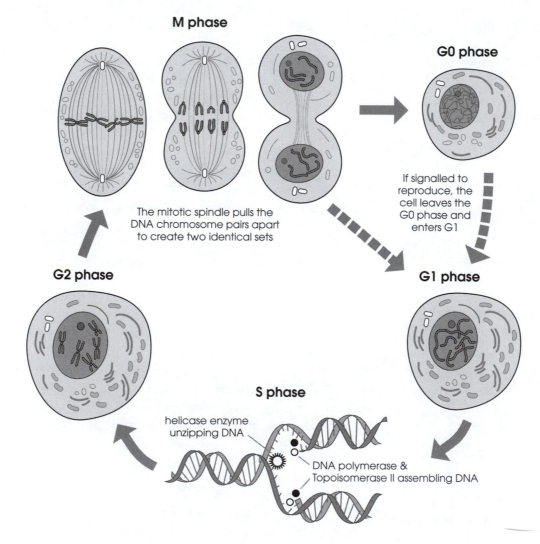

The cell cycle

Let's look at the cell cycle phases in more detail:

GI Phase (Gap I)

During the G1 phase the cell begins to produce the components needed for two cells. It grows in size, stores energy, and increases production of RNA and the proteins necessary for DNA formation. This stage is also considered to be an important checkpoint. The cell biologically monitors all of its components as well as its size and internal environment. If it is not ready for the DNA duplication process of the next stage, the cell goes into a growth and repair (G0) phase.

S Phase (Synthesis)

This is the phase in which the cell's DNA is duplicated in preparation for mitosis. DNA duplication is a very precise, complex, and energy consuming process. Specific enzymes and proteins are involved, some already having been made in G1 and some synthesized during this phase.

The DNA structure is a double helix – double-stranded with a helix or coiled shape. Before the actual duplication process can begin, the DNA must untwist or unwind itself to become two straight single strands. The enzyme helicase 'unzips' the DNA, following which several other enzymes including DNA polymerase and topoisomerase II ensure that the strands replicate properly.

At the end of DNA duplication the cell enters another G phase.

G2 Phase (Gap 2)

During G2 the cell continues to grow, produces new proteins, and stores more energy in preparation for division. In addition to a double volume of DNA, by the end of this phase it contains all the substances needed for two cells. This phase also serves as another important checkpoint for the cell. The new DNA is evaluated for proper duplication and the other cellular components are checked to ensure they are ready for the next process.

M Phase (Mitosis)

Mitosis, or cell division, occurs during this phase. Mitosis takes place over several stages that culminate in the separation of the cellular components into two identical daughter cells. Integral to this process is the formation of the mitotic spindle, a specialized biological structure that only forms when cells are dividing. The spindle consists of a series of protein (tubulin) microtubules that facilitate the separation of DNA chromosomes in opposite directions to ensure that each new cell has its own complete set of DNA.

G0 (Zero) Phase

After cell division has occurred and two daughter cells are formed, the new cells can either re-enter the replication cycle or go into a G0 (non-reproductive) state. Cells in G0 perform their normal metabolic functions, but otherwise cellular activity during this phase is considerably less than during the reproductive cycle.

Most cells in the body are in a G0 state, carrying on with normal cellular functions. However, labile cells in structures like the GI tract, skin, bone marrow, and hair follicles are continuously re-entering the replication cycle. In this way they are somewhat similar to the rapidly reproducing cells of cancerous growths, and as a result they are more vulnerable to the effects of anti-cancer drugs than other types of normal body cells.

Drugs Used in Cancer Treatment

The cancer patient is usually taking several types of medications. Some are specific cancer fighting drugs while others are used to combat treatment side effects, pain, nutritional deficiencies, anxiety, depression, and so on. Many of these adjunctive use medications have been addressed in earlier chapters, for example analgesics in Chapter 6, anti-anxiety and antidepressant drugs in Chapter 10, and medications for stabilizing cardiovascular function in Chapter 7. The massage therapist must be prepared to investigate the diverse drug combinations clients with cancer may be using.

In this chapter the focus is on two groups of pharmaceuticals:

- the antineoplastic drugs
- antinausea or antiemetic drugs

1.   THE ANTINEOPLASTIC DRUGS

The antineoplastics work in a variety of ways to either destroy cancer cells or disrupt tumors. They include:

- drugs that affect cell replication
- drugs that affect tumor growth

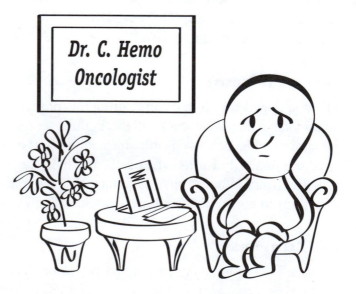

Dr. C. Hemo
Oncologist

Drugs that Affect Cell Replication

This category encompasses several different types of medications:

- alkylating drugs
- antimetabolites
- antitumor antibiotics
- drugs that affect the mitotic spindle

- **alkylating drugs**

The commonly used alkylating drugs are: busulfan (Myleran), mechlorethamine (Mustargen, Nitrogen Mustard), chlorambucil (Leukeran), cyclophosphamide (Cytoxan, Neosar), and dacarbazine (DTIC-Dome).

Mechanism of Action

This drug group is widely used in chemotherapy. They are described as 'cell proliferation dependent but cell-cycle phase nonspecific,' meaning that they can be effective during any phase of the cell cycle.

However, the alkylating drugs are most proficient at influencing the S phase. They form crosslinks between the two strands of the double helixed DNA and prevent it from unzipping and unwinding. The DNA becomes unable to duplicate, and enzymes, proteins, and other cellular components cannot be synthesized. Cellular metabolism and reproduction are compromised and the cell eventually dies.

- **antimetabolites**

The most frequently prescribed drugs in this category include: fludarabine (FLUDARA), methotrexate (Folex, Mexate), fluorouracil (Adrucil), floxuridine (FUDR), and cytarabine (Cytosar-U).

Mechanism of Action

The antimetabolite group consists of several substances that are similar in structure to normal intracellular elements and can compete with them in various ways. Like the alkylating drugs, the antimetabolites can produce effects during all phases of the cell cycle but are most effective during the S phase.

RNA and DNA synthesis are the processes primarily targeted. For example, methotrexate and fluorouracil are directly inserted into DNA and RNA components or compete for receptor sites on enzymes to disrupt their activities. The end result is formation of defective strands of RNA and DNA and reduced cell replication.

Folic acid and thymidylate are examples of essential substances used by cells in the production of DNA and RNA. Methotrexate is described as a folic acid antagonist because it interferes with the biochemical transformation of folic acid. Fluorouracil, on the other hand, seems to disrupt thymidylate.

The antimetabolites are quite sensitive to the most rapidly dividing cells in the body, which include cancer cells, bone marrow, skin, intestinal mucosa, and urinary bladder cells.

- **antitumor antibiotics**

Names of drugs in this category include: actinomycin D (Dactinomycin), daunorubicin (Daunomycin, Cerubidine), doxorubicin (Adriamycin), idarubicin (Idamycin), bleomycin (Blenoxane), and plicamycin (Mithracin).

Mechanism of Action

These drugs are antibiotics that have been found to have cancer-fighting properties. They can affect cells during any part of the cell cycle and are used either alone or in combination with other antineoplastic drugs.

The mechanisms of action of the antitumor antibiotics are not completely understood. They appear to interact with DNA in a variety of ways. Their methods include:

- disrupting the interaction between DNA and the enzyme RNA polymerase

- binding to DNA and preventing unwinding of the double helix

- inhibiting the function of the topoisomerase II enzyme, resulting in production of DNA strands that are likely to cleave and break

- **drugs that affect the mitotic spindle**

The commonly prescribed drugs in this group are: paclitaxel (Taxol), vincristine (Oncovin, Vincasar), and vinblastine (Velban, Velsar).

Mechanism of Action

These drugs are also known as the **tubulin inhibitors**. They act specifically to impair cell division by influencing the formation and/or breakdown of the mitotic spindle during the M phase of the cell cycle. The result is that the spindle is not effective in separating the DNA chromosomes into two sets. Without successful completion of DNA duplication, the cell will not reproduce.

Drugs that Affect Tumor Growth

Pharmaceuticals that perform functions to discourage tumor growth include:

- hormonal agents
- interferons
- angiogenesis inhibitors

- **hormonal agents**

Hormonal agents are used to address cancers whose tumor growth is dependent in some way on hormones.

Mechanism of Action

These drugs either block hormone receptor sites on tumors or influence the body's production of hormones on which tumors are dependent. The hormones usually associated with tumor growth are the male and female sex hormones testosterone and estrogen. For example, metastatic prostate cancer is testosterone dependent and most breast cancers show estrogen dependency. Luteinizing hormone, produced in the pituitary gland, can also play a role in tumor growth.

Tumors that are androgen (testosterone) dependent can be treated with estrogenic hormones to antagonize the actions of testosterone, while estrogen dependent cancers can be treated with androgenic hormones.

Hormones like the corticosteroids are used to treat lymphoid tumors because of their specific catabolic effect on lymphatic tissues.

Antiestrogenic Drugs: Drugs such as tamoxifen (Novaldex) and toremifene (Fareston) are relatively new antiestrogen agents. Some cancers, for example a number of breast cancer types, have estrogen receptors on their cells. Estrogen stimulation causes such tumors to enlarge. Tamoxifen is believed to act by blocking these estrogen receptors. Another drug that has an effect on estrogen is anastrozole (Arimidex). It inhibits the enzyme aromatase, which is found in breast, muscle, liver, and adipose tissues. Aromatase plays an important role in the formation of estrone, an estrogen precursor. Many types of breast cancer cells also contain aromatase and therefore seem able to make their own estrogen. By inhibiting the actions of aromatase, anastrozole is able to reduce the concentration of circulating estrogen and discourage tumor growth.

Antiandrogenic Drugs: Antiandrogenic drugs such as flutamide (Euflex, Eulexin), nilutamide (Nilandron), and bicalutamide (Casodex), used in the treatment of prostatic cancer, block testosterone receptors on the prostate. Another antiandrogenic mechanism of action is to decrease circulating levels of testosterone by affecting the biochemical chain of events culminating in testosterone production and release.

How LHRH Analogs Affect Circulating Testosterone

The hypothalamus regulates the plasma testosterone level. If the volume of circulating testosterone drops, the hypothalamus produces luteinizing hormone-releasing hormone (LHRH) which stimulates the pituitary gland to release luteinizing hormone (LH) and adrenocorticotropic hormone (ACTH). LH stimulates the testes, which produce about 90% of circulating testosterone; ACTH stimulates the adrenal glands, which also produce and release some testosterone. When the plasma testosterone level is high, this information is relayed to the hypothalamus via a negative feedback loop and it decreases its production of LHRH.

The drugs goserelin (Zoladex, Zoladex LA) and buserelin (Suprefact) are known as LHRH analogs. These drugs mimic the actions of naturally produced LHRH. Research shows that when LHRH is continuously released the initial result is increased LH and testosterone levels. However, constant stimulation leads to the pituitary becoming desensitized to the effects of LHRH and production of testosterone begins to drop. The LHRH analogs can produce this effect.

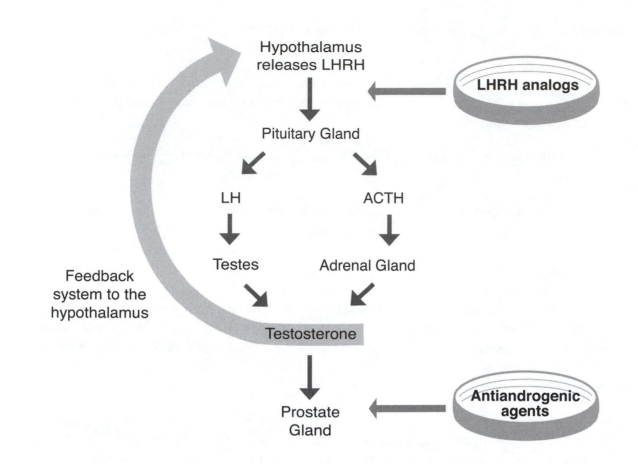

- **interferons**

Interferons are naturally occurring compounds produced by cells in response to stimuli like viruses, tumors, and foreign substances that cause antibody production. Pharmaceutical forms include: interferon beta-1b (Betaseron), interferon-alpha (Veldona), and interferon alfa-2a (Intron A).

Mechanism of Action

How interferons work is still not fully understood, but immune system cells such as natural T killers and the macrophages involved in recognizing and eliminating tumor cells seem to be activated by them.

The human body produces three types of interferons:

- interferon alpha, produced by leukocytes and lymphoblastoid cells when stimulated by viruses and other cell irritants

- interferon beta, primarily produced by fibroblasts

- interferon gamma, also known as immune interferon, produced by T lymphocytes in response to antigenic and mitogenic (induces cell mitosis) stimulation

As a group these interferons perform the following functions:

- stimulate healthy cells to resist infection
- protect cells against viral infections
- inhibit the growth of some cells, in particular cancer cells
- modify immune system responses as needed

The last two functions are particularly important in resisting tumor growth.

- **angiogenesis inhibitors**

The angiogenesis inhibitors are a very new category of drugs that are bringing fresh hope to the fight against cancer. Still undergoing clinical trials (over 100 drugs are presently being tested[7]), these pharmaceuticals disrupt the formation of blood vessels to tumors.

Mechanism of Action

Angiogenesis, the formation of blood vessels to match blood supply needs, is essential to the growth and development of any tissue or organ. Tumors are no different. A solid tumor can only grow to the size of a pinhead (1-2 cubic millimeters) before it needs to start attracting new blood vessel branches in order to meet its nutritional requirements. Tumors produce factors such as Tumor Angiogenesis Factor (TAF) to induce blood vessels to connect to them. The new angiogenesis inhibitors are being designed to block or inhibit these factors in various ways.

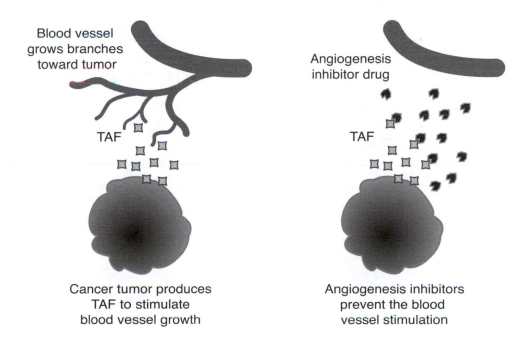

Cancer tumor produces TAF to stimulate blood vessel growth

Angiogenesis inhibitors prevent the blood vessel stimulation

Because of the mechanism of action of these drugs, they are not expected to cause side effects like the gastrointestinal irritation, bone marrow suppression, and hair loss associated with many of the chemotherapeutic agents. It is too early to know which drugs in this category will be the most effective and what types of side effects they may cause.

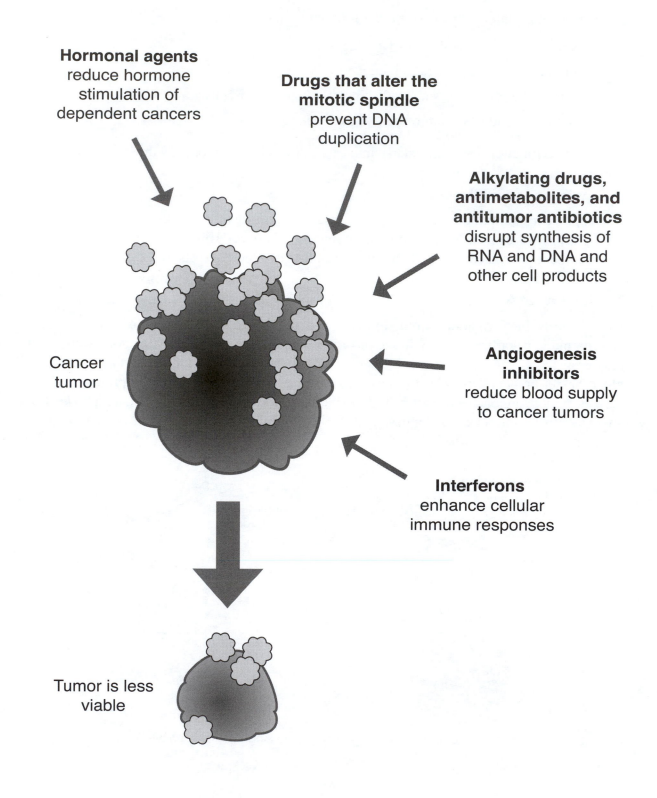

Actions of the antineoplastic drugs

2.   THE ANTINAUSEA OR ANTI-EMETIC DRUGS

Commonly prescribed medications in this group include: dolasetron mesylate (Anzemet), odansetron (Zofran ODT), granisetron hydrochloride (Kytril), dexamethasone (Decadron), diphenhydramine (Benadryl), and prochlorperazine (Compazine).

Nausea and vomiting, sometimes quite severe, are experienced by many cancer patients. They result from:

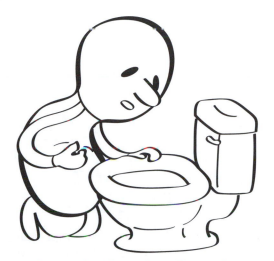

- specific cancer types and locations, e.g. stomach and pancreatic cancers

- a number of antineoplastic pharmaceuticals

- radiation of sites like the liver and GI tract

The sensation of nausea and the act of vomiting are the result of a series of neural messages and reflexes involving various systems. The final control signal comes from the vomiting center located in the medulla of the brainstem. In addition to the vomiting center, some of the structures involved include:

- the chemoreceptor trigger zone (CTZ)

- the vestibular apparatus (involved in motion sickness)

- the respiratory center

- receptors located in the stomach, small intestines, and pharynx

Nausea and vomiting can result in dehydration, electrolyte imbalance, and loss of interest in eating. The patient can become very debilitated at a time when nutrition and good sleep are important. The negative anticipation of feeling sick can be psychologically distressing in itself for people entering cancer treatment. Management of nausea and vomiting, preferably prophylactically, has become an important aspect of cancer care.

Drugs that are used in the treatment of nausea and vomiting act in various locations, including:

- the vestibular apparatus (antihistamines)

- the GI tract (metoclopramide)

- the CTZ (phenothiazines, metoclopramide)

- a variety of receptor sites (antihistamines, odansetron, granisetron)

The Common Anti-Emetic Drugs

DRUG	MECHANISM OF ACTION	SIDE EFFECTS
Scopolamine (Transderm ScÇp) Dimenhydrinate (Dramamine) Meclizine (Antivert, Bonine) Hydroxyzine (Atarax, Vistaril)	These drugs occupy histamine and cholinergic receptor sites in the vestibular area.	Refer to the information about antihistamines in Chapter 9.
Metoclopramide (Reglan)	This drug can block dopamine and serotonin receptor sites. It reduces stimulation of the CTZ and increases normal emptying of the stomach and GI tract.	Very similar to the phenothiazines. Refer to Chapter 10.
Chlorpromazine (Thorazine) Prochlorperazine (Compazine) Thiethylperazine (Torecan) Perphenazine (Trilafon) Haloperidol (Haldol) Droperidol (Inapsine)	These drugs act within the CTZ to occupy/block dopamine receptor sites.	Refer to the information about phenothiazines in Chapter 10.
Dexamethasone (Decadron)	This drug's exact mechanism of action in achieving its anti-emetic effects is not known. Often used in combination with other drugs.	Belongs to the corticosteroid group. Refer to Chapter 6.
Ondansetron (Zofran) Granisetron (Kytril)	These drugs, called the selective 5-HT3 inhibitors, occupy/block specific serotonin receptor sites in the stomach, on the vagus nerve, in the CTZ, and in an area called the solitary tract nucleus.	Headaches, malaise, fatigue, constipation, diarrhea, abdominal pain, weakness, anxiety, dry mouth, dizziness, shivers, hypotension, skin rash.

SIDE EFFECTS – Drugs for Managing Cancer

This table lists the common side effects of the groups of medications discussed in this chapter. Therapists must keep in mind that other side effects may occur, and that reactions will vary in degree and intensity. Always ask clients about incidence and intensity of any side effects experienced. When more than one medication is being taken, whether in the same drug group or not, therapists should appreciate the increased potential for adverse and idiosyncratic effects.

Side Effects	AD	AM	ATA	HA	MSD	IF	Side Effects	AD	AM	ATA	HA	MSD	IF
Abdominal Pain		X	XX			X	Breathing Difficulties			XX			
Anaphylaxis			XXX				Cardiotoxicity	XXX		XX			
Anemia	XX	XX	XXX	X	XXX		Chest Pains				XX		XX
Anorexia	XX	XX	XX	XX	XX	XX	Chills		X	X			
Anxiety						X	CNS Depression					XX	
Blood Disorders	XXX	XXX	XXX	XXX	XXX		Confusion		X				
Blurred Vision				X		X	Constipation					X	X
Bone Pain			xxx(t)				Convulsions	XXX	XXX			XXX	
Bradycardia				X			Cramps		XX				

Side Effects	AD	AM	ATA	HA	MSD	IF
Cranial Nerve Paralysis					XX	
Cystitis				xxx(f)		
Decreased Reflexes					XX	
Deep Vein Thrombosis				xxx(t)		
Depression				X	X	X
Dermatitis	X	X				
Diarrhea	XX		XX	X	XX	XX
Dizziness	X			X		XX
Drowsiness				X		
Dry Skin		X				
Earache						X
Ecchymosis		X				
Edema				xx(f)		
Endometrial Cancer				xxx(t)		
Electrolyte Changes	XX					
Fatigue		X		X		X
Fever		X	X			X
Folliculitis		X	X			
Granulocytopenia						XX
Gastritis		X				
GI Bleeding		XXX			XX	
Gynecomastia	X			xxx(f)		
Hair Loss	X	X	X	X	X	X
Headaches	X	X		X		X
Hearing Loss	XX					
Hemiparesis		XX				
Hepatitis				xxx(f)		
Hot Flashes				X		
Hypercalcemia				xxx(t)		
Hyperpigmentation	X	X				
Hypertension		XX		xx(f)		
Hypotension			XX	XXX	X	
Impotence		X		X		
Insomnia						XX
Irritability						X
Irritated Injection Site				xx(f)		
Increased Bleeding					XX	
Joint Pain				X		X
Kidney Toxicity	XXX	XXX		XXX	XXX	
Leukopenia	XXX	XX	XXX	XXX	XXX	XXX

Side Effects	AD	AM	ATA	HA	MSD	IF
Lightheadedness				xx(t)		
Liver Toxicity	XXX	XXX	XXX	XXX	XXX	
Menstrual Irregularities	X	X		xxx(t)		
Mood Changes				X		XX
Myalgia		X			X	X
Myelosuppression	XXX	XX			XXX	
Nausea	X	X	X	X	X	XX
Nervousness						X
Numbness					XX	
Orthostatic Hypertension		XX				
Orthostatic Hypotension					XX	
Paralytic Ileum					XXX	
Pelvic Pain				xxx(t)		
Peripheral Edema				xxx(t)		
Peripheral Neuropathy	X				XX	X
Photosensitivity		X		xx(f)	X	
Pneumonia			XX			
Prickling Skin Sensation	X				X	X
Pulmonary Embolism				xxx(t)		
Pulmonary Fibrosis	XXX		XXX		XXX	
Rectal Bleeding				xxx(f)		
Respiratory Congestion						X
Rhinitis						X
Rigors						X
Seizures					XXX	
Skin Rash	XX	XX	XX	XX	XX	X
Spermatogenesis Chgs		X				
Sterility	X					
Stomach Pain		X	XX		X	
Stroke				xxx(t)		
Tachycardia				XX	XX	
Taste Changes				X		X
Thrombocytopenia	XXX	XXX	XXX	XXX	XXX	XX
Tinnitus	X					X
Ulcers		X				
Vaginal Bleeding				xxx(t)		
Vomiting	X		X	X	X	XX
Weakness					XX	X
Weight Loss	XX		XX			
Wheezing					XX	

AD: Alkylating Drugs, AM: Antimetabolites, ATA: Antitumor Antibiotics, HA: Hormonal Agents, MSD: Mitotic Spindle Drugs, IF: Interferons

(t) relates specifically to the antiestrogenic drugs, eg. tamoxifen

(f) relates specifically to the antiandrogenic drugs, eg. flutamide

X – tolerable – notify medical practitioner if bothersome

XX – serious – monitor closely and notify medical practitioner

XXX – very serious – seek medical attention as soon as possible

Quick Guide to Case History Taking for Clients Who Have Cancer

It can be challenging to put together a treatment plan that takes into account the many factors involved in cancer scenarios. The reader is referred to *Massage Therapy and Cancer*[8] by Debra Curties. This text explores in more detail the clinical decision-making issues for massage therapists working with clients who have cancer.

Questions

1. What type of cancer is it? Date diagnosed? Known metastases?

2. How has it been treated so far? Surgery? Radiation? Drug therapies? What is the present treatment protocol? Any alternative therapies being used? (Be prepared to research.)

3. If surgery has been done, ask about:
   * which tissues/organs were involved, what was removed (including lymph nodes)
   * date of the procedure(s)
   * post-surgical recovery – any setbacks, delayed healing, infections?
   * present condition of the area, quality of repair, how well remaining tissues are functioning; altered sensation, edema, decreased r.o.m., other complications?
   * location of the scar(s) and current state (numb, hypersensitive?), client's comfort level with having them seen/touched

4. If radiation has been done, ascertain when and where, the current state of integrity of the skin and underlying structures, and whether the affected area has altered sensation. If the client is in the middle of a radiation protocol, clarify what the schedule is. Check on the current condition of the site(s) and the presence of 'exit' burns. Ask about any medical restrictions placed on touch, temperature exposure, and lubrication use.

5. Get details about drug therapy: protocol (drugs being used, schedule), side effects, condition of skin, joints, and other connective tissues, any ongoing effects from prior chemotherapy.

6. Inquire about body system function, blood pressure fluctuations, and presence of any systemic disorders. If present, how are they being managed?

7. Is the client in pain? If yes, ask about the nature and behavior of the pain, severity on a pain scale. How is the pain level affected by being touched?

8. Skin irritations, infections, or rashes? Open sores or other lesions? Easy bruising? Get details about locations, causes. Any problems with healing delays?

9. How is the client's energy level? How does it fluctuate with the treatment protocol?

10. Support system – family, friends, health care team, support group? Does the client feel well supported?

11. Stress levels, stress management strategies? Problems with anxiety, depression? If yes, how managed?

12. Experience with massage therapy? What are the client's goals in receiving massage?

Observations

1. Assess the general posture of the client. Antalgic postures? Protective holding patterns? Disability adjustments?

2. Observe skin color, signs of health and vitality. Observe any skin lesions present. Any radiation marks or tattoos?

3. Check scars and treatment areas for tissue integrity, sensation status. (Proceed at the client's comfort level.)

4. Check for edema. If present, is it pitted?

Quick Guide to Working with Clients Who Have Cancer

Cancer symptoms, treatment protocol 'on' and 'off' phases, and medication side effects can cause day-to-day physical and emotional state fluctuations. Before each treatment ensure you are familiar with the client's current health status and energy level. Be flexible in adjusting your approach to the circumstances and the client's goals for each session.

1. Pay particular attention to the health of the skin and underlying tissues. Radiation treatment, chemotherapy effects, and the disease progression can alter the health and sensitivity of all body tissue types. It is easy to cause injury with approaches that are too aggressive. Clearly identify areas of sensory loss or impairment. Begin cautiously, adjusting the depth, pressure, and rate and rhythm of your techniques as appropriate. Communicate regularly to get information from the client about how the treatment feels, but be aware that you cannot entirely rely on the accuracy of this feedback.

2. Cancer effects and cancer therapies can greatly tax the liver, heart, and kidneys. Keep current on the status of these systems and any therapies being used to support their function. Modify your treatment approach accordingly.

3. Adjust your appointment schedule to be compatible with the client's chemotherapy and radiation protocols and the resulting fluctuations in physical health, mood, and stamina. It is generally best to wait after 'therapy days' to give the client recovery time – a day or two is typical but the time needed often gets longer as the client proceeds with the protocol. Comply with medical directives about touch, hygiene, and lubrication for recent radiation burns. Never blur or 'erase' ink markings for radiation sites.

4. Begin with shorter, lighter treatments. Evaluate responses to therapy closely with the client. Consult with the medical team if you need guidance in designing an appropriate treatment plan.

5. Be prepared for the fact that massage treatment may not always be appropriate. If the client seems too unwell or has developed new symptoms that have not yet been medically evaluated, postpone the session. Make sure the client knows that he or she can cancel at short notice if not feeling up to receiving massage.

6. Position for comfort. Use pillows, towels, bolsters, and blankets to ensure optimal ease and adequate support, especially if the client is in pain, has range of motion limitations, or is very thin (cachexic). Ensure that affected limbs or body areas are positioned safely – do not place undue stress on recent surgery or radiation sites.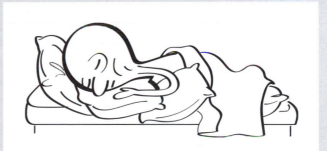

7. Choose approaches and techniques that focus on relaxation. Clients undergoing cancer treatment are usually stressed, tense, and anxious. They often need to feel nurtured and to re-experience a sense of physical enjoyment. Relaxation also helps to increase the immune fighting ability of the body and reduce nausea. Encourage deep breathing, however exercise caution with clients who are respiration compromised.

General Guidelines

1.   Keep track of the medications and remedies, prescribed or otherwise, that the client is taking. Inquire routinely about medication type and dosage changes. The client will often be using pharmaceuticals in addition to anticancer drugs. These could include, for example, anti-anxiety medications, corticosteroids, narcotic analgesics, or antibiotics. Many of these drug groups have been discussed in previous chapters of this book, but others have not. Therapists are encouraged to refer to a drug reference text or to research on the Internet to obtain needed information about client medications.

2.   Peripheral neuropathy, joint and muscle pain, and muscle atrophy and weakness are often side effects of chemotherapy. Changes in soft tissue health, for example inflammation, irritation, fragility, poor healing, bruising, and altered sensation are also common. A medical opinion is often necessary to determine whether such symptoms are related to drug side effects.

3.   Chemotherapy can cause liver and kidney toxicity disorders. Accumulation of the drugs and their metabolites can leave the client's body in a weakened state. Normal performance of liver and kidney functions is also affected and clients can develop secondary symptomology like hypertension, CHF, respiratory congestion, peripheral edema, and jaundice. Do not hesitate to postpone sessions and refer for medical evaluation. When massage is appropriate, shorter lighter treatments are recommended.

4.   The anticancer drugs suppress the immune system in several ways, resulting in increased susceptibility to infections and more difficulty fighting them off. Routine hygienic practices are especially important for practitioners working with clients who have cancer. If the person becomes ill with an infection or develops a fever, massage is not recommended until the condition has subsided. If you yourself are ill, avoid risking infecting the client by rescheduling for a later date.

5.   Cardiovascular and blood disorder concerns such as chest pains, blood pressure changes, cardiotoxicity, dysrhythmia, anemia, and bone marrow suppression are all side effects of the antineoplastic drugs. Monitor the client's blood pressure on an ongoing basis and be alert to changes or complaints of a cardiovascular nature. Blood disorders can predispose the client to bleeding/bruising and require modification of manual techniques. Refer to Chapter 7 for more about CV system related guidelines.

6.   Orthostatic hypotension, dizziness, and lightheadedness are side effects of several of the medications used. These symptoms can be intensified after a massage treatment. Give clear instructions concerning getting on and off the table – determine if the client needs help.

7.   Dehydration, poor nutritional status, and electrolyte loss from gastrointestinal irritation are often due to the effects of chemotherapy. Such clients will have low energy and will fatigue quickly. Be prepared to shorten your treatment time and keep in mind that tissues can be more easily irritated or injured if aggressive manual techniques are used. Light rhythmic stroking on the back can help reduce nausea and gastrointestinal upset.[8]

8.   Skin hypersensitivity, rashes, and photosensitivity reactions can occur with several of the anticancer drugs. The skin is easily inflamed or injured. Modify technique pressures. Do not massage on-site where there is a skin rash or local inflammation.

9.   Modify appropriately around injection sites and implanted medication delivery devices. Guidelines related to this subject are addressed in detail in Chapter 5.

Specific Guidelines

1.   Alkylating Drugs

Use of these drugs often causes respiratory system compromise (pulmonary fibrosis), increasing the workload of the muscles of respiration. It is a good idea to incorporate more focus on these muscles, as appropriate, in your treatment plan. In addition, poor oxygen delivery and inadequate carbon dioxide removal can weaken body tissues. Stay alert about the depth of your manual techniques.

Convulsions and seizures can occur as central nervous system side effects of this drug group. Consult to evaluate whether massage therapy is appropriate for the client. If massage is approved, determine what treatment scheduling is best suited to the stability of the condition.

Peripheral neuropathy may also occur. The symptoms can vary tremendously in degree and intensity. Identify exactly where the areas of involvement are. If the symptoms are severe, avoid local massage; if the problem is more mild, employ light techniques and monitor how the client's body responds. Keep in mind that sensory perception may be altered.

2.   Antimetabolites

These drugs are associated with a number of CV and blood disorders, including easy bleeding, slow clotting, increased blood pressure, and anemia. It is important to adjust the depth of your manual techniques as a matter of course when the antimetabolites are being used. Monitor cardiovascular changes on a treatment by treatment basis.

The information about central and peripheral nervous system side effects presented in the section above for the alkylating drugs applies as well to the antimetabolite group.

3.   **Antitumor Antibiotics**

The antitumor antibiotics produce respiratory side effects as outlined for the alkylating drugs, and their potential blood and cardiovascular complications are the same as those described above for the antimetabolites.

4.   **Hormonal Agents**

Tamoxifen use is related to increased incidence of deep vein thrombosis (DVT), which often presents as complaints of calf and foot muscle cramping, tired feet, and swollen ankles. Local massage where a thrombus is present can result in serious complications. If suspicious, refer for medical evaluation before massaging the affected body part.

Irritated injection sites are typical of flutamide. Evaluate the site carefully and refer to Chapter 5 for treatment related guidelines.

The information given about blood and cardiovascular side effects in the antimetabolite section applies to the hormonal agents as a group. In addition, orthostatic hypotension is very commonly reported with these drugs.

5.   **Drugs that Affect the Mitotic Spindle**

Like the alkylating drug group and the antitumor antibiotics, mitotic spindle drugs can cause pulmonary fibrosis. Check the information given earlier in these Specific Guidelines. Similarly, seizures, convulsions, and peripheral neuropathies can occur with use of drugs in this category.

Specific to this group of anticancer medications is a complication called paralytic ileus (intestinal paralysis) that can lead to bowel obstruction. Presence of symptoms that may be indicating this condition, such as constipation, pain, and increasing distension should be treated as a medical emergency. Massage treatment is contraindicated.

6.   **Interferons**

Interferon use can cause insomnia and mood changes. It is important to be sensitive to the fact that emotional symptoms may be beyond the client's control. Shorter treatments may be appropriate.

Hydrotherapy Guidelines

Clients taking antineoplastic drugs and various adjunctive medications can pose a number of concerns related to hydrotherapy use. Before making any hydrotherapy decisions, confirm whether there are medically prescribed temperature or modality restrictions and check on the presence of sensory changes or impairments. Take note of all the medications being used and how they could influence hydrotherapy effects.

Cardiovascular Concerns: Heart and blood vessel responses are altered by many of the drugs a client with cancer might be taking. Blood vessels may overreact to mild stimuli and produce adverse effects like vasospasm and vascular pooling. Easy bleeding and slower clotting can be exacerbated by hydrotherapy applications. The heart, liver, and kidneys under stress frequently react adversely to intense stimuli like systemic hydrotherapy. Systemic treatments should be modified or eliminated from the treatment plan altogether when the vital organ systems are compromised.

Respiratory Concerns: Steams, saunas, and other forms of systemic hydrotherapy that increase respiratory workload are not recommended. This is especially true for clients with pulmonary fibrosis or who complain of shortness of breath.

General Enervation: The fatigued or debilitated client is more likely to benefit from smaller local applications with modified temperatures.

Tissue Sensitivities: Chemotherapy and radiation treatments can make the skin and underlying tissues fragile and either hypersensitive or hyposensitive to temperature stimuli. As a general rule, it is contraindicated to wet rashes or other open sores or skin lesions. There are usually specific restrictions placed on water applications at radiation sites.

Inquire about the bath or shower practices used at home or by the hospital/hospice staff – this information is a guide to what is being well tolerated. If in doubt, seek medical advice. Where it is considered appropriate, introduce hydrotherapy slowly and incrementally into the treatment plan. Ensure that other members of the health care team are aware of your program and that it is compatible with the rest of the client's treatment schedule.

Vomiting and diarrhea stress the abdominal musculature. Cool abdominal washes support the general health of the gastrointestinal tract and relieve muscle soreness. However, abdominal hydrotherapy is contraindicated with gastrointestinal bleeding or severe irritation or restriction in bowel function.

Dehydration is a common result of GI disturbances – encourage adequate hydration, especially when using heat modalities.

Exercise Recommendation

Build your exercise plan around the client's lifestyle, energy level, and body system health. Ensure that there is medical approval for any exercise program being undertaken. Consult with other members of the health care team if uncertain about how specific activities might affect the medical treatment protocol or cancer progression. Monitor closely.

Make sure the client is aware of the importance of adequate hydration and nutrition before and during exercise.

Be alert to complaints of cramps, extremity swelling, and muscle fatigue. These may be related to a serious complaint like deep vein thrombosis. Medical evaluation is important to assess for this complication – exercise must be suspended until the 'all clear' is given. These symptoms may also be more minor medication side effects or caused by low electrolyte levels. In this case, modified exercise may still be appropriate.

Some of the drugs used for managing cancer can predispose to photosensitivity reactions. Instruct such clients to avoid exercising in direct sunlight.

Any respiratory or cardiovascular disorders or other major health status concerns must be taken into account. The client's current activity level can be a useful guide in designing an exercise plan. However, do not exceed your scope of practice. It is important to acknowledge when greater expertise is required.

1. The National Cancer Institute of Canada, "Current Incidence and Mortality" www.cancer.ca/stats/highle.htm

2. Fierro, M., "How Much Does Cancer Cost?" *Health Policy Studies* www.nga.org/center/divisions/1,1188,T_CEN_HES%5EC_ISSUE_BRIEF%5ED_1915,00.html

3. Margaret Foti, Ph.D, American Association for Cancer Research, "Defeating Cancer - A Sense of Urgency and a Need for Strategic Continuity," *Testimony before the House Appropriations Subcommittee on Labor, Health and Human Services, Education,* March 21, 2000. www.aacr.org/5000/5300/5300e.html

4. B.C. Cancer Agency, *Cancer in General*, revised April 2001 www.bccancer.bc.ca/pg_t_03.asp?PageID=8&ParentID=2

5. "Chemotherapy and You. A Guide to Self Help During Cancer Treatment," *NIH Publication,* revised June 1999, (99): 1136, National Cancer Institute cancernet.nci.nih.gov/peb/chemo_you/index.html

6. Cancer Liaison Program, Office of Special Health Issues, Office of International and Constituents Relations, U.S. Food and Drug Administration www.fda.gov/oashi/cancer/cdrugind.html

7. "Review of Anti-Angiogenesis Drugs for Lung Cancer" www.lungcancerclaims.com/antiangiogenis%20lung%20cancer.htm

8. Curties, D., *Massage Therapy & Cancer*, Curties-Overzet Publications, Moncton, 1999

CHAPTER 12

Drugs for Managing HIV/AIDS

Since its discovery almost twenty years ago the human immunodeficiency virus (HIV), the organism that causes AIDS, has challenged scientists and researchers to find a cure. The urgency to solve the mysteries of AIDS and find a vaccine or drug that can eliminate it is fueled by the tremendous toll this disease is taking globally:[1]

- As of the end of 2000, an estimated 36.1 million people worldwide (34.7 million adults and 1.4 million children under 15) were living with HIV/AIDS.

- Approximately 5.3 million new HIV infections (about 15,000 per day) occurred during 2000.

- The year 2000's global mortality rate was approximately 3 million people, including an estimated 500,000 children under 15.

North American statistics include the following information:

- The Centers for Disease Control and Prevention (CDC) estimate that 800,000 to 900,000 U.S. residents are living with HIV, one-third of whom are unaware of their infection.

- Approximately 40,000 new HIV infections occur each year in the United States, 70% in men and 30% in women. Half of the newly infected people are under 25.

- As of the end of 2000, a total of 774,467 cases of AIDS in the U.S. population had been reported to the CDC and 448,060 deaths had been recorded. AIDS is now the fifth leading cause of death in the United States.

- A cumulative total of 45,534 positive HIV tests were reported in Canada[2] up to December 31, 1999.

Viruses are especially difficult to counteract because they incorporate themselves into the host body's own cells. The majority, however, like the measles and mumps viruses, are self-limiting in most people. The appearance of HIV has motivated researchers to focus with greater intensity on developing effective antiviral drugs. It is a painstaking and expensive process – the average cost of researching and developing a single drug for human use is about $500 million. One company reportedly spent more than $1 billion over a ten-year period to develop a protease inhibitor. There are currently 78 pharmaceutical and biotechnology companies researching and developing over 113 antiviral medicines and vaccines.[3]

Despite the fact that there is still no cure for HIV/AIDS, important advances have resulted in the development of a number of medications that significantly extend life expectancy for people who test HIV positive. In order to understand how they work, it is necessary to consider the structure and replication cycle of the virus.

Viral Structure

A virus is one of the smallest living microorganisms. It consists of strands of DNA or RNA (the viral genetic code) contained inside a shell called a capsid or nucleocapsid. A glycoprotein envelope, actually made from a small section of the prior host cell's membrane, surrounds and protects the capsid and its viral core material. Protruding though this envelope are spiky extensions that help the virus detect and attach to cellular receptor proteins.

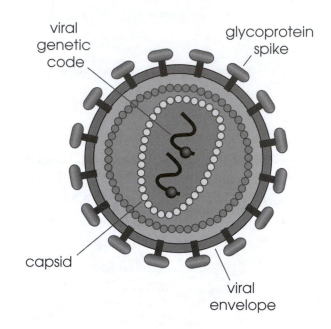

Viruses such as the chicken pox and herpes simplex viruses contain DNA, while those with RNA strands, such as measles and HIV, are known as **retroviruses**.

Replication Cycle of a Virus

Once established in a host, a single virus can produce more than one billion new viruses per day. This is typical production for HIV, even though each virus only lives about 1.6 days. There are several steps or phases[4] in viral replication, including:

- binding
- entry
- uncoating and reverse transcription
- nuclear entry
- integration and transcription
- translation, assembly, and budding

We will examine these steps in more detail using the specific example of the HIV retrovirus.

Phase 1: Binding

The HIV virus is attracted to T helper cells, which are immune cells that play an important role in the body's defense against invading organisms and foreign substances. These cells have a marker or receptor called CD4 on their surfaces. When the virus identifies a cell with CD4 receptors it attaches itself to the cell's membrane.

Phase 2: Entry

The virus then penetrates the host cell and squeezes its capsid through the cell's membrane and into the cytoplasm. All the substances necessary for viral replication, including several forms of its RNA and the enzymes reverse transcriptase, integrase, and protease, are included in the material inserted into the cell.

Phase 3: Uncoating and Reverse Transcription

Once inside the cell the capsid opens and releases its contents directly into the cytoplasm. Using the enzyme reverse transcriptase, the virus begins to transcribe its RNA genetic code into a form that resembles the DNA of the host cell. This is necessary because the cell's nucleus will only allow entry to DNA.

Phase 4: Nuclear Entry

Once the virus has made its own form of DNA the strands are transported to the host cell's nucleus where they are allowed easy access through the nuclear membrane.

Phase 5: Integration and Transcription

Inside the nucleus the virus uses the enzyme integrase to insert its own genetic material into the host cell's DNA. The viral DNA, with all the mechanisms for self-replication in place, can remain dormant within the host cell nucleus for months or years before it is activated. Once activated, the virus takes control of the cell and begins its replication process. It starts by re-converting its DNA into viral RNA, which leaves the nucleus and re-enters the cell's cytoplasm.

Phase 6: Translation, Assembly, and Budding

The viral RNA is 'translated' into long bands or chains of viral proteins, which are then cut into smaller pieces by the enzyme protease. The resulting genetic parts are assembled by messenger RNA into numerous sets of core viral material resembling the contents of the virus that originally infected the cell.

Once assembled the viral particles migrate in groups to the cell membrane. In order to be able to infect other cells this viral material must leave the host cell and enter the blood. Each set of viral core material pushes into the cell membrane to form a 'bud' which eventually breaks away from the cell. As it does so it takes a piece of the cell membrane with it, forming an external envelope for the new virus.

An infected host cell can produce millions of viral copies before its resources are exhausted and it dies.

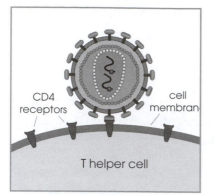

Phase 1: attraction

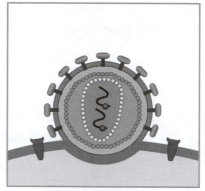

Phase 1: binding

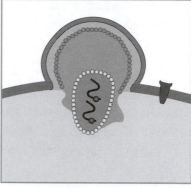

Phase 2: entry

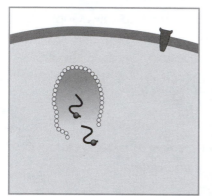

Phase 3: uncoating

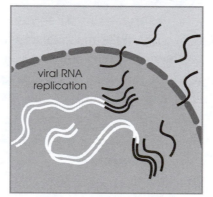

Phase 3: reverse transcription

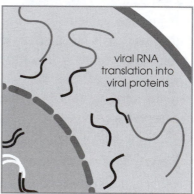

Phase 4: nuclear entry

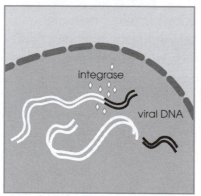

Phase 4: integration

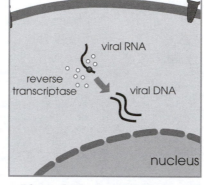

Phase 4: transcription

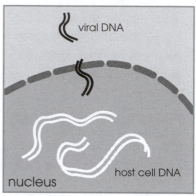

Phase 5: translation

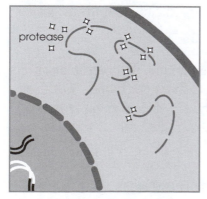

Phase 5: assembly

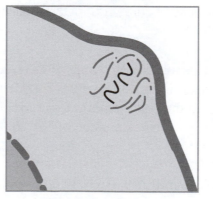

Phase 6: budding

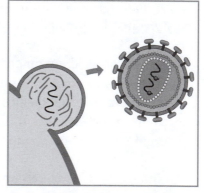

Phase 6: release

1.   ANTIVIRAL DRUGS

Antiviral drugs act to disrupt enzyme functions at several stages of the viral replication process. Where possible these drugs are designed to target the specific characteristics and behaviors of individual viruses, as is the goal with HIV. HIV pharmaceutical treatment protocols are often referred to as 'drug cocktails,' since several drugs are used in combination.

This chapter will focus on the following drug groups:

- reverse transcriptase inhibitors
  - nucleoside analogues reverse transcriptase inhibitors (NRTIs)
  - non-nucleoside reverse transcriptase inhibitors (NNRTIs)
- protease inhibitors
- interferons
- new drugs under development

Nucleoside Analogues Reverse Transcriptase Inhibitors (NRTIs)

Drugs in this category include: AZT, zidovudine (Retrovir), acyclovir (Zovirax), ddI, didanosine (Videx), ddC, zalcitabine (Hivid), d4T, stavudine (Zerit), and 3TC, lamivudine (Epivir).

AZT, which was approved in 1987, was the first official anti-AIDS drug. Prior to that acyclovir had been approved in 1982 for treating herpes infections in hospitalized patients with compromised immune systems. These two drugs, and the other members of the NRTI group, are now commonly used in combination with other antiviral medications in the overall management of HIV and AIDS-related diseases.

Mechanism of Action

Nucleotides are the bases, or building blocks, of DNA and RNA. There are five nucleotides: adenosine (adenine), cytidine (cytosine), guanosine (guanine), thymidine (thymine), and uridine (uracil). They combine in specific pairs and with other compounds to form either DNA (deoxyribonucleic acid), or RNA (ribonucleic acid).

During the uncoating and reverse transcription phase of viral replication, the virus converts its own RNA structure into DNA strands. The viral DNA is accepted by the host cell's nucleus in part because the enzyme reverse transcriptase utilizes the cell's own stored nucleotides to assemble its strands.

The term analogue is used in chemistry to denote compounds that are structurally similar. Nucleosides are components of nucleotides (a nucleoside + phosphoric acid = a nucleotide). The NRTIs are nucleoside-like compounds that enter body cells and are incorporated by intracellular enzymatic processes into forms that resemble normal nucleotides. Reverse transcriptase begins to use these 'false' nucleotides to form viral DNA strands. The result is defective DNA that cannot be integrated into the host cell DNA, inhibiting or slowing down the replication process.

A serious side effect of the NRTIs is lactic acidosis.[5] It is a complication that can make the person extremely ill, but the onset is often not distinguished quickly enough from the general AIDS-related symptom picture. The signs and symptoms of lactic acidosis include:

nausea and vomiting

abdominal pain

liver dysfunction

anorexia and weight loss

lethargy and general malaise

hyperventilation and/or dyspnea

cardiac dysrhythmia

cyanosis and cold extremities

Non-Nucleoside Reverse Transcriptase Inhibitors (NNRTIs)

In 1996, nevirapine (Viramune) was the first member of this drug group to be granted accelerated approval by the Food and Drug Administration. Others include delavirdine (Rescriptor) and efavirenz (Sustiva). The NNRTIs are also used in combination with other antiviral drugs to control HIV/AIDS.

Mechanism of Action

The NNRTIs disrupt the formation of viral DNA, but they use a different mechanism from the NRTIs. They inhibit the activities of reverse transcriptase by binding onto it. Without this enzyme the virus is unable to make its DNA, and the replication process comes to a halt.

Peripheral neuropathy is a commonly experienced side effect of the NNRTIs. It occurs in varying degrees of intensity and at its most severe is very painful. Symptoms include numbness and tingling, reduced reflexes at the ankle, and aching/burning pain in the legs and feet that can be intense enough to prevent walking. There may also be signs of nerve inflammation and muscle atrophy.

Protease Inhibitors (PIs)

This group of drugs, which includes amprenavir (Agenerase), saquinavir (Fortovase), ritonavir (Norvir), indinavir (Crixivan), nelfinavir (Viracept), and lopinavir/ritonavir (Kaletra), was first introduced in late 1995. They are much more powerful than the reverse transcriptase inhibitors and have been rapidly incorporated into the drug cocktails used to manage HIV/AIDS. As of 1999 their global market value was already estimated at approximately $2 billion.[6]

Mechanism of Action

The antiviral activity of the protease inhibitors occurs during the translation, assembly, and budding phase of viral replication. They interfere with the role played by the protease enzyme, which cuts long chains of proteins into smaller sections of viral core material.

The protease inhibitors resemble viral protein chains. They put themselves in the way of the protease enzyme, causing it to cut the drug instead of the viral strands. The ensuing process of assembling units of genetic material incorporates improperly cut viral strands; the new viruses that are ultimately produced are defective and non-infectious.

Lipodystrophy, a disturbance or defect of fat metabolism, is often observed in protease inhibitor users. Fat is typically lost from the arms, legs, and face, and appears to be redistributed around the abdomen and at the cervicothoracic junction, where it forms a 'buffalo hump.' The exact cause of this metabolic change is not clear and is currently being researched.

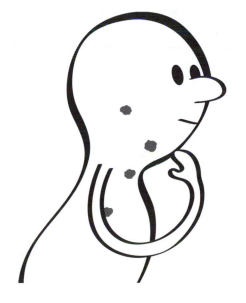

Interferons

Interferons are released from lymphocytes, macrophages, fibroblasts, and certain types of epithelia following viral exposure. Their purpose is to stimulate non-infected cells to produce antiviral substances to protect themselves from attack.

Interferons also assist in controlling cell growth and replication, which has led to their role in cancer therapy. In addition to their antiviral properties, interferons are used in the HIV context to treat Kaposi's sarcoma, a blood vessel cancer closely associated with AIDS.

For more information, the reader is referred to the section about interferons in Chapter 11.

New Drugs Under Development

The drugs presently in use to manage viral infections all affect the virus's replication process once it is inside a host cell. New antiretroviral drugs currently in clinical trials, called the 'entry inhibitors,' seem to be able to prevent the virus from binding to and entering cells.[7]

Second generation protease inhibitors[8] are also under investigation. They have an improved chemical structure that allows for better antiviral activity. Laboratory testing shows encouraging results against the HIV virus, but these drugs have not yet entered the clinical trial phase.

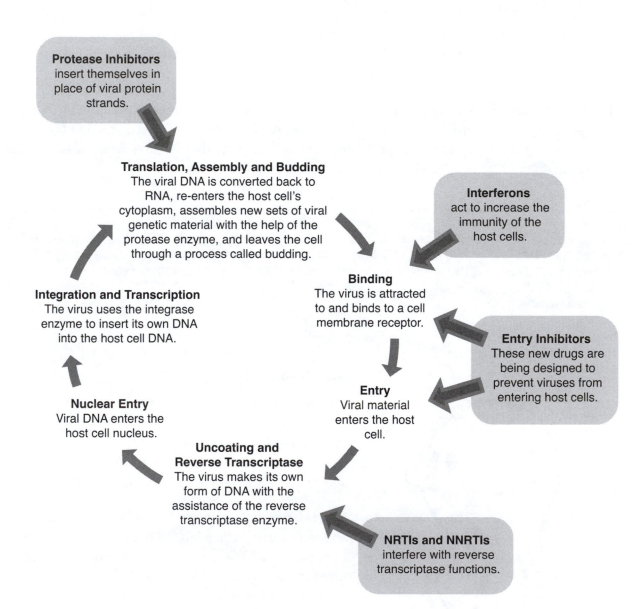

The actions of the antiviral drugs

SIDE EFFECTS – Drugs for Managing HIV/AIDS

This table lists the common side effects of the groups of medications discussed in this chapter. Therapists must keep in mind that other side effects may occur, and that reactions will vary in degree and intensity. Always ask clients about incidence and intensity of any side effects experienced. When more than one medication is being taken, whether in the same drug group or not, therapists should appreciate the increased potential for adverse and idiosyncratic effects.

Side Effects	PI	NRTI	NNRTI
Abdominal Pain	X		X
Anemia	XX	XX	XX
Anorexia	X		X
Anxiety	X		X
Arthritis	X	X	
Ataxia	X		
Back Pain	X		
Blood Disorders	XXX	XXX	XXX
Blurred Vision	X	X	
Bacterial, Viral, Fungal Infections	XX		
Breast Enlargement	X		
Chest Pain	XX		
Chills	X	X	X
CNS Depression		XX	XXX
Confusion	X	X	
Convulsions	XXX	XXX	
Cough	X	X	
Cramps	X		
Decreased Concentration			XX
Depression	X		XX
Diarrhea	XX	X	XXX
Dizziness	X	X	XX
Dreams – Intense, Unusual	X		XX
Dry Mouth	X	X	
Dyspepsia		X	
Edema	X		
Euphoria	X		
Ear Pain	X	X	
Face, Tooth Pain	X		
Fat Redistribution	XX		
Fatigue, Drowsiness	X	X	XX
Fever	XX	X	X
GI Distress, Constipation	XX	X	X
Hair Loss	X	X	
Hyperesthesia	XX		
Hyperglycemia	XX		
Hyper/Hyporeflexia	X		
Headaches		XX	XXX
Hypertension	X	XX	
Hypotension	X		

Side Effects	PI	NRTI	NNRTI
Increased Bleeding	X	XXX	
Increased Cholesterol, Triglycerides	XXX	XX	XX
Insomnia	X	X	XXX
Intense And Unusual Dreams	X		XX
Kidney Stones	X		
Lactic Acidosis		XXX	
Leukopenia	XX		XX
Libido Disorders	X		
Liver Disorders	XXX	XXX	XXX
Menstrual Irregularities	X		
Microhemorrhages	XX		
Mood Changes			X
Mouth Sores		XX	
Muscle Atrophy	X	XX	
Myalgia	X	X	X
Nausea	XX	XX	XX
Nervousness	X	X	
Neutropenia	XXX	XXX	XXX
Nosebleeds		X	
Palpitations	XX	XX	
Pancreatitis	XX	XXX	XXX
Peripheral Neuropathy	XXX	XXX	XXX
Photosensitivity	X		
Pneumonia	XX	XX	
Prickling Skin Sensation	XX		
Psychotic Disorder	X		
Respiratory Disorder	XX	XX	
Rhinitis	X		
Seizures	XXX	XXX	
Skin Rash	XX	XX	XX
Skin Ulcers And Other Changes	XX		
Splenomegaly	XX		
Sweating	X	X	
Swollen Belly	XX		
Taste Changes	X	X	XX
Thrombocytopenia	XX		XX
Vasodilation		XX	
Vomiting	X		X
Weakness	X	XX	X
Weight Increase/Loss	XX		

NA: Nucleoside Analogues, NNRTI: Non-Nucleoside Reverse Transcriptase Inhibitors, PI: Protease Inhibitors

x – tolerable – notify medical practitioner if bothersome

xx – serious – monitor closely and notify medical practitioner

xxx – very serious – seek medical attention

Quick Guide to Case History Questions

HIV positive clients have health statuses that range from normal health through terminal illness, so case history taking needs to reflect the circumstances in each case. Most people with HIV/AIDS are educated about their condition - don't hesitate to ask questions.

Questions

1. Date of HIV diagnosis; stage and progression. History of related illness? Is the condition presently well stabilized? If the person has active AIDS, get details of current symptom picture, opportunistic conditions.

2. Medications: identify all pharmaceuticals and remedies being used. Is the drug cocktail working well? Ask about medication side effects – how are they being addressed? Have there been any episodes of drug toxicity, especially recently? If yes, how managed?

3. Method(s) of medication administration – any injection sites or implanted devices?

4. Vital system health: Inquire about the status of the heart, liver, and kidneys in particular, as well as presence of any systemic disorders. Any problems with blood pressure control? If yes, how managed? Any breathing difficulties?

5. General nutritional status: Eating properly – good appetite? Taking nutritional supplements? Ask about current or recent experience of anorexia, nausea, vomiting, diarrhea, or constipation (contribute to dehydration, electrolyte loss, decreased absorption of nutrients). Any recent unexplained changes in weight? General tissue health, healing times?

6. Inquire in detail about skin health – rashes, irritated areas, locations of hypo- or hypersensitivity, open lesions, skin cancers. Any topical medication applications?

7. Success with handling stress? Problems with anxiety, depression? If yes, how managed?

8. Support system – family, friends, health care team, support group? Does the client feel well supported?

9. Experience with massage? Goals in seeking out massage therapy?

Observations

1. Observe general posture, body weight/thinness, gait and mobility, breathing patterns.

2. Check the skin for:
   - color and signs of vitality
   - texture and moisture
   - rashes, infections, lesions
   - scars: identify relevance - related to lesion removal, injection sites?
   - fragility, discoloration, bruising

3. Edema – if present, check for pitting.

4. Observe any locations of altered tissue sensation.

5. Check for fatty tissue redistribution.

Quick Guide to General Treatment Issues with HIV/AIDS Clients

Medication side effects and AIDS-related symptoms can vary from one session to the next. Ensure you are familiar with the client's current health picture before beginning each treatment. Be flexible in adjusting your approach to the circumstances and the client's goals.

1. Familiarize yourself with the universal AIDS prevention guidelines, which should form the basis of your hygienic practices with **all** clients. You can obtain these documents by contacting the National AIDS Information Clearinghouse (1-800-458-5231) or the AIDS Hotline (1-800-342-2437), or view them at the Centers for Disease Control and Prevention website: www.cdc.gov/ncidod/hip/blood/universa.htm. A good Canadian source is the Canadian HIV/AIDS Clearinghouse (1-877-999-7740), website: www.clearinghouse.cpha.ca.

   Find answers to any questions you may have about the spread of HIV, as well as guidelines for health care workers.

2. Remember that clients with AIDS have compromised immune systems. If you are ill with anything contagious, postpone the appointment. Be conscientious about infection control in your treatment space, especially if an earlier client has had a 'bug.'

3. Begin slowly with new clients and monitor responses to therapy closely. If unsure about treatment plan decisions, consult with the attending physician.

4. Take the client's blood pressure regularly. It is good clinical practice and helps to monitor cardiovascular stress and medication side effects. Pre- and post-treatment blood pressures can also help you evaluate the response to therapy.

5. Adapt your treatment plan around tissue fragility and sensory changes. Local treatment is contraindicated where there are skin rashes or lesions.

6. Client position and comfort: Some HIV/AIDS clients will have painful musculoskeletal symptoms – positioning needs to be adapted to what is comfortable. Keep the room warm and use blankets as needed – chills and cold extremities can affect the client's comfort and ability to relax during the treatment. The cachexic client must be well pillowed to avoid pressure on bony prominences.

Choice of Techniques

1. Maintain a strong focus on relaxation. Encourage deep and relaxed breathing, especially at the start of treatments (adapt if there are respiratory complications).

2. When edema is present, elevate the tissues/limbs to facilitate drainage. Exercise appropriate precautions if the cardiovascular system is weakened (see Chapter 7).

3. Modified effleurage and petrissage, slow rhythmic techniques, passive range of motion, and gentle joint play are usually appropriate for clients who have more advanced AIDS illnesses.

4. Deep and aggressive techniques are not recommended where there is tissue fragility or impaired sensation.

General Guidelines

1. Clients with HIV/AIDS can be taking several types of drugs for various reasons, including:

    •   managing the HIV virus (the drug cocktail)

    •   controlling/preventing a variety of medication side effects

    •   treating AIDS-related diseases/conditions like pneumocystis carini, candidiasis, and other fungal infections, tuberculosis, Kaposi's sarcoma, dementia, and cytomegalovirus infections such as hepatitis, pneumonia, retinitis, and colitis

    In addition, supplements, herbs, and remedies are often used.

    Some of the adjunctive medications a client with HIV can be taking will have been discussed in previous chapters of this book while others will not. Be prepared to research in drug reference texts or on the Internet.

    Multiple medication use, especially with some of the potent pharmaceuticals in drug cocktails, can predispose to adverse and toxic effects. Practitioners should always be vigilant in monitoring changes in client signs and symptoms.

2. There are some severe side effects common to the drugs discussed in this chapter. The ones that follow usually contraindicate massage therapy until they have been medically addressed and stabilized:

    •   **pancreatitis:** Early indicators of pancreatitis can be overlooked among the general medication side effects and symptoms of the disease. Be alert to complaints of nausea, vomiting, and abdominal pain that refers to the back.

    •   **blood disorders:** Thrombocytopenia, leukopenia, neutropenia, and severe anemia are examples of the more serious blood disorders that can develop. If the person has been medically evaluated and massage is appropriate, the practitioner must pay careful attention to the health of the tissues and to microvasculature fragility. Deep or aggressive techniques are contraindicated.

    •   **liver dysfunction:** The liver's normal physiologic functions are often suppressed or impaired by medication effects, and liver dysfunction in turn contributes to poor metabolism and excretion of drugs. Toxic metabolite accumulation can occur and produce adverse reactions.

    •   **skin rashes and irritations:** Skin lesions of varying degrees of seriousness can develop for a number of reasons in the AIDS client. In some cases, especially when there is a rapid acute onset, a skin rash may be indicating a severe drug reaction. Another possibility is the development of a secondary infection like shingles. These can be very serious in immunocompromised individuals.

3. Be sensitive to the client's health changes from treatment to treatment. Anorexia, vomiting, diarrhea, and liver and blood disorders occur frequently with antiretroviral medications. Their effects can be quite enervating, causing weakness and debilitation that can be made worse by massage and hydrotherapy treatments that are too intense. Make sure that the client knows it is okay to cancel appointments, even on short notice, if he or she is feeling too unwell.

4. Musculoskeletal aches and pains are common complaints associated with taking HIV/AIDS medications. Given all the factors, related or unrelated to HIV, that may cause this type of symptom, it can be difficult to discern whether the complaints are medication side effects. If massage work is not proving effective, or if the practitioner senses that the symptoms are not 'routine,' medical follow-up should occur.

5. Peripheral neuropathy can be caused by progression of the AIDS condition or by an AIDS-related infection, or it can be a drug-induced side effect. The intensity of peripheral neuropathy symptoms varies considerably – at its most severe it may make touch intolerable. If massage is indicated, aspects of the treatment plan like client positioning and technique depth will need to be modified. Keep in mind that client feedback will likely be inaccurate.

6. Facial pain, ear pain, and headaches are all common side effects of the medications discussed in this chapter. Inquire about the most comfortable position(s) and pillow for protection and support.

7. Because of medication effects like dizziness, fatigue, and orthostatic hypotension, give clear instructions concerning getting on and off the massage table – help the client if necessary.

8. Some clients will have implanted medication delivery devices. Ensure that such devices are not compromised by the client's position. For more detailed guidelines, refer to Chapter 5.

Specific Guidelines

1. Nucleoside Analogues Reverse Transcriptase Inhibitors (NRTIs)

Lactic acidosis can be a serious side effect of this medication group. Massage therapy is contraindicated until the condition is resolved. Practitioners should be vigilant for lactic acidosis symptoms (listed earlier in this chapter). If a client appears to be developing this condition, advise immediate medical care.

Some people develop breathing problems like asthma. Check for respiratory system medications (refer to Chapter 9). It may be appropriate to focus additional attention on treating the muscles of respiration.

The NRTIs are associated with easy bleeding. Observe for signs of bruising and make sure to modify technique depth as a matter of course with clients using medications in this group.

Vasodilation, caused by skeletal muscle atrophy (resulting in reduced vein support), can lead to the development of extremity edema. Observe for varicosities, and exercise caution when working around distended veins. Position the edematous tissues to facilitate drainage. Refer to Chapters 5 and 7 for more guidelines related to peripheral vasodilation.

The NRTIs often cause hypertension, which will be controlled medically as much as possible by altering the antiviral drug mix and adding antihypertensives. There is the potential, however, for chronic hypertension to stress the heart and promote a degree of heart failure. If this is the case, the massage therapist needs to incorporate treatment adaptations as outlined in Chapter 7.

Central nervous system depression may be present, causing generalized fatigue that may necessitate shorter treatments. The implications of CNS depression for massage treatment planning are discussed in more detail in Chapter 10.

Seizures and convulsions also occur in some people. If the condition has been stabilized and massage therapy is considered appropriate, schedule your sessions in order to maximize bioavailability of the anticonvulsant medications.

2. **Non-Nucleoside Reverse Transcriptase Inhibitors (NNRTIs)**

Central nervous system side effects like dizziness, headaches, depression, poor concentration, and insomnia are associated with NNRTI use. These effects tend to occur for a few weeks following start of therapy. Clients are more easily overtaxed physically and emotionally. It is important to be sensitive and flexible. Shift to a shorter, less intense treatment design.

Gastrointestinal distress, especially diarrhea, can be a problem with the NNRTIs. If not properly managed, it can lead to a degree of electrolyte loss that predisposes to cardiac dysrhythmia. As well, muscles and their tendons can become hyper-responsive to manual techniques, resulting in cramping and spasms. It is important for the client to maintain hydration and good nutrition, and to seek medical assistance with diarrhea control. The massage therapist may need to restrict technique usage to very light, rhythmical approaches.

3. **Protease Inhibitors (PIs)**

Kidney stones can develop when these drugs are used. The initial symptom is usually sharp cramping pain, often referred to as flank pain, that is experienced in the vicinity of the kidney and down the lateral back deep into the abdomen. The pain may also spread to the groin. A complaint of this nature should be referred to the physician.

Lipodystrophy is associated with protease inhibitor use. The client may not notice these changes immediately, especially if they occur on the back. If this is the case, bring it to the client's attention and suggest medical follow up. When massaging, be aware of the possible sensitivity of the affected tissues and modify your manual techniques accordingly. Any aggressive approach to 'break up' lipid accumulations is contraindicated.

Hyperglycemia, believed to be related to the fatty tissue redistribution, can be a problem, especially for diabetics. If you perceive that this side effect may be developing, suggest follow-up medical evaluation. If the client is or has become diabetic, the massage therapy treatment design needs to be adapted to be compatible with diabetic stability. Signs and symptoms of hyperglycemia, as well as treatment issues and medications for diabetes, are discussed in Chapter 8.

When increased skin sensitivity or other tissue hyperesthesias are present, manual techniques need to be carefully modified. Identify the affected tissue locations and adjust technique rate and depth to the specific circumstance. In severe cases touch may not be tolerable either locally or generally.

Some individuals experience microhemorrhaging when taking protease inhibitors. Be alert for bruising and modify manual techniques around affected tissue areas.

Hydrotherapy Guidelines

Hydrotherapy helps strengthen the body physiologically; utilized appropriately it can be an important part of massage treatment protocols for clients with HIV. Proceed cautiously, beginning with mild applications that are well tolerated and monitoring reactions to treatment carefully.

Always determine whether medical restrictions have been placed on temperature use or on the wetting of any skin surfaces, and identify locations of altered sensation. If uncertain, discuss the proposed procedure with the physician.

Peripheral neuropathy and tissue hyperesthesia can be aggravated by hydrotherapy applications. Inquire about the client's routine bath/shower temperatures and use this information as a guide in treatment planning.

The PIs and NRTIs can cause increased sweating, especially with systemic heat exposure. If the client is experiencing this side effect, inquire about whether he or she is drinking fluids and replacing electrolytes. This information will help the therapist gauge the appropriateness of heat applications. In general, hot systemic modalities are not likely to be advisable.

Systemic hot hydrotherapy can also intensify the vasodilation effects associated with NRTI medications and adverse reactions such as dizziness and lightheadedness can occur. Systemic heat should be avoided unless the client assures you that hot baths/showers are well tolerated. Some local modalities, like hot footbaths, can also increase vasodilation significantly. With local treatments, precautions would include using reduced temperatures, smaller applications, and shortened treatment times. Always monitor the client's reactions carefully.

> Cool abdominal washes are effective in strengthening and toning the digestive tract; warm footbaths can reduce insomnia; and cool compresses to the neck often alleviate headaches. Used in a gentle progressive manner such modalities may help manage drug-related side effects.

Exercise Recommendation

Design your exercise plan around the client's usual activity and energy levels. Consult with members of the health care team if unsure about how your proposed exercise program might impact on the client's health.

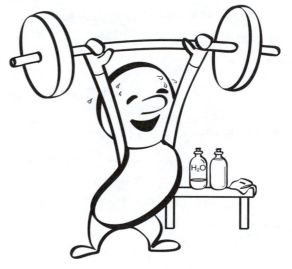

Increased sweating, a side effect of the protease inhibitors and NRTIs, can lead to dehydration and electrolyte imbalance. This is a particular concern if the client is exercising in hot/humid conditions. Episodes of diarrhea and vomiting can also cause dehydration and electrolyte deficiency. Remind the client of the importance of good nutrition and fluid replacement before and during exercise.

Photosensitivity reactions sometimes occur with protease inhibitor use. When exercising outdoors the person should be well clothed and perform activities in shaded areas.

Fatigue and weakness, peripheral neuropathy, and muscle and joint pain are all medication side effects that can alter the HIV/AIDS client's ability to exercise. Make sure that the intensity, frequency, and duration of the suggested exercises are reasonable in each client's case. Re-evaluate the exercise plan if the client complains of symptom intensification.

1. Office of Communications and Public Liaison, National Institute of Allergy and Infectious Diseases, National Institutes of Health, "HIV/AIDS Statistics Worldwide," *MD Public Health Service*, U.S. Department of Health and Human Services, August 2001 www.niaid.nih.gov/factsheets/aidsstat.htm

2. Division of HIV/AIDS Surveillance, Bureau of HIV/AIDS, STD and TB Laboratory Centre for Disease Control, Health Protection Branch Health Canada, "Reported AIDS Diagnoses," *HIV and AIDS in Canada Surveillance Report to December 31, 1999* www.avert.org/canstatg.htm

3. Pharmaceutical Research and Manufacturers of America, *AIDS and The Pharmaceutical Industry*, Washington, DC www.phrma.org/publications/backgrounders/development/aids98.phtml

4. "Retroviral Reproduction," *ARIC's On-Line AIDS Medical Glossary* www.critpath.org/aric/gloss/body/retroviral_reproduction.htm

5. Shikuma, C., "What is Lactic Acidosis Syndrome and Mitochondrial Toxicity?" National AIDS Treatment Advocacy Project (NATAP), University of Hawaii www.natap.org/2000/lipo/lipo_rp4pt1whatislact092200.htm

6. *HIV/AIDS, Pipeline & Products*, Vertex Pharmaceuticals www.vpharm.com/NonEnhanced/AntiviralNonE.html

7. Blakeslee, D.J., "Entry Inhibitors: The More the Better," *JAMA HIV AIDS Resource Center*, September 22, 2000 www.ama-assn.org/special/hiv/newsline/conferen/icaac00/dbentry.htm

8. "Adding to Antiretroviral Arsenal: New AIDS Drugs in Development. Resistance Repellant?" *CBS HealthWatch*, February, 2001 cbshealthwatch.medscape.com/cx/viewarticle/234098_3

Bibliography

Website References

Pain and Inflammation

Harris, M., "The Treatment of Spasticity: As Difficult as it is Diverse," Adorno Rogers Technology, Inc., *Website Content*, 2000 http://www.artmobility.com/community/features/f-spasticity_03_28.htm

The Life Extension Foundation, "Acetaminophen Poisoning (Analgesic Toxicity)," *Website Content*, 2000 www.lef.org/protocols/prtcl-001.shtml

National Institute of Neurological Disorders and Stroke (NINDS), "NINDS Spasticity Information Page," *Website Content*, 2001 www.ninds.nih.gov/health_and_medical/disorders/spasticity_doc.htm

Cardiovascular

American Heart Association, "2001 Heart and Stroke Statistical Update," *Website Content*, 2001 www.americanhea.org/statistics/pdf/HSSTATS2001_1.0.pdf

American Heart Association, "Cardiovascular Disease Statistic," *Website Content*, 2000 www.americanheart.org/Heart_and_Stroke_A_Z_Guide/cvds.html

Bandolier Evidence Based Healthcare, "Calcium Channel Blockers and Hypertension," *Website Content,* October 1995 www.jr2.ox.ac.uk/bandolier/band20/b20-1.html

Cardiovascular Consultants Medical Group, "Calcium Channel Blockers," *Website Content*, 2001 www.healthyhearts.com/ccb.htm

Desai, U.R., "Cardiac Glycosides," *Lecture*, School of Pharmacy, Virginia Commonwealth University, 2000 www.people.vcu.edu/~urdesai/car.htm

ExRx: Fitness Testing, "Blood Cholesterol," *Website Content*, 2001 www.exrx.net/Testing/CholScreen.html

Hass, E.M., "Vitamin K," excerpt, Staying Healthy with Nutrition: The Complete Guide to Diet and Nutritional Medicine, *Website Content*, HealthWorld Online, 2001 www.healthy.net/asp/templates/article.asp?PageType=article&ID=2140

Health Central, "Hyperlipidemia: Acquired," *Website Content*, 2001 www.healthcentral.com/mhc/top/000403.cfm?src=ls

Humana, "Management of Hyperlipidlemia," *Website Content*, 2001 www.humana.com/providers/guidelines/hyperlip.asp

Piepho, R.W., "Pharmacology of The Calcium Channel Blockers," *Article*, Emory University, Atlanta, 2001 www.emory.edu/WHSC/MED/CME/CCB/toc.html

The University of Utah, NetPharmacology, "Cardiovascular Pharmacology," *Lecture Notes*, 2000 www.lysine.pharm.utah.edu/netpharm/netpharm_00/notes.html

Diabetes

ALtruis Biomedical Network, "Diabetes-Drugs.net," *Website Content*, 2000-01 www.diabetes-drugs.net

American Academy of Family Physicians, "Diabetes: How to Use Insulin," *Website Content*, 1999 www.aafp.org/afp/990800ap/990800i.html

American Diabetes Association, *Website Content*, 2001 www.diabetes.org/main/application/commercewf

AutoControl Medical, *Website Content*, 2001 www.autocontrol.com

Bristol-Myers Squibb Company, New Jersey, "Oral Medications – Biguanides," *Website Content*, 2001 www.glucovance.com/treatment/biguanides.html

Diabetes Home, "Types of Insulin," *Website Content*, 2001 www.diabeteshome.ca/pages/types-of-insulin.html

Diabetes Insight, "Insulin Onset, Peak Activity and Duration Chart," *Website Content*, 2000 www.diabetic.org.uk/lwd/management/medication/insulin_2001.htm

Disetronic, "Pump Therapy: Choosing Control," *Website Content*, 2001 www.disetronic-usa.com

Ixion, "The Cost of Care," *Website Content*, 2001 www.ixion-biotech.com/diamkt.htm

Joslin Diabetes Center, "A Few Facts About Diabetes," *Website Content*, 2001 www.joslin.harvard.edu/education/library/wfewfact.html

Lawson, M.L., "Insulin Pump Therapy: Is it Right for You?" *Diabetes Dialogue*, Winter 2000, Canadian Diabetes Ass'n www.diabetes.ca/membership/dialogue/win00-insulinpump.html

Lifeclinic.com, "Medications for Diabetes," *Website Content*, 2000 www.lifeclinic.com/focus/diabetes/Insulin_types.asp

National Diabetes Information Clearinghouse, "Medicines for People with Diabetes," *Website Content*, 2000 www.niddk.nih.gov/health/diabetes/pubs/med/index.htm

"Scientists in New Insulin Pump Hope for Diabetes" *Birmingham Post News Digest*, February 28, 2000, *Adicol Website Content* www.adicol.org/mix/public_index.htm

Siu-Chan, W., "Information about Insulin," the Daily Apple, *Website Content,* 2000 www.thedailyapple.com/target/cs/article/tda/100868.html

Respiratory

American Lung Association, "Asthma," *Website Content*, 2001 www.lungusa.org/asthma

American Lung Association, "Trends In Asthma Morbidity and Mortality, January 2001," *Website Content*, 2001 www.lungusa.org/data/asthma/asthmach_1.html#economic

American Lung Association, "Estimated Prevalence of Lung Disease," Lung Association Report, April 2001 www.lungusa.org/data/lae_01/lae.html#bronchitis

Asthma and Allergy Foundation of America (AAFA), Asthma and Allergy Information, "Asthma Facts," *Website Content*, 2001   www.aafa.org/asthmaandallergyinformation/ aboutasthmaandallergies/factsandfigures/asthma_facts.cfm

Doctor's Guide Publishing Limited, "FDA Approves Xopenex For Bronchospasm Treatment," *Website Content*, 1999 asthma.about.com/gi/dynamic/offsite.htm?site=http:// www.pslgroup.com/dg/efd9a.htm

Medscape Resource Center, "Asthma Diagnosis and Treatment," Medscape Inc., *Website Content*, 2001 www.medscape.com/Medscape/features/ResourceCenter/ Asthma/public/RC-index-Asthma.html

United States Environmental Protection Agency, "Asthma and Upper Respiratory Illness," *Website Content*, 2001 http://www.epa.gov/children/asthma.htm

Mood and Emotional Disorders

Agency for Health Care Policy and Research (AHCPR), "Depression is a Treatable Illness: A Patient's Guide," *Website Content*   www.mentalhealth.com/bookah/p44-dp.html

Anxiety Disorders Association of America, "Misdiagnosis of Anxiety Disorders Costs U.S. Billions," *Website Content*, 1999 http://panicdisorder.about.com/gi/dynamic/offsite.htm?site=http ://www.adaa.org/dyna/view.cfm%3FID=5

Department of Psychiatry, Washington University St. Louis, "Depression Facts," *Website Content*, 2001 www.psychiatry.wustl.edu/depression/depression_facts.htm

"Depression: A Global, National and Personal Burden," *Website Content* www.depression_resources.ofinterest.com/depression/article.htm

National Institute of Mental Health, "Anxiety Disorders," *Website Content*   www.nimh.nih.gov/anxiety/anxiety/idx_fax.htm#top

Screening for Mental Health Inc., "Depression: Frequently Asked Questions," *Website Content*, 2001 www.nmisp.org/dep/depfaq.htm

Stephens, T., Joubert, N., "The Economic Burden of Mental Health Problems in Canada," *Chronic Diseases in Canada*, 22(1), 2001, Mental Health Promotion Unit of Health Canada www.hc_sc.gc.ca/hpb/lcdc/publicat/cdic/cdic221/cd221d_e.html

SANE, "Medical Methods of Treatment," *Website Content*, 2001 www.sane.org.uk/About_Mental_Illness/Medical_Treatments.htm

"The Neurobiology of Depression," *Website Content*, www.depression-resources.ofinterest.com/neurobiology/article.htm

The Schizophrenia Homepage, "U.S. Health Official Puts Schizophrenia Costs at $65 billion," *Website Content*, 1996 www.schizophrenia.com/news/costs1.html

The University of Texas, Addiction Science Research and Education Center, College of Pharmacy, "Dopamine, A Sample Neurotransmitter," *Website Content*, 2001 www.utexas.edu/research/asrec/dopamine.html

Vernon, R.F., "Antidepressants Made Easy: An Introduction to Tricyclics and Selective Serotonin Re-Uptake Inhibitors," University of Southern California, 1997 www-scf.usc.edu/~rvernon/antidepressants.html

Frederickson, A., "The Dopamine Hypothesis of Schizophrenia," Serendip *Website Content*, 1998 www.serendip.brynmawr.edu/bb/neuro/neuro98/ 202s98-paper2/Frederickson2.html

Cancer

B.C. Cancer Agency Care and Research, "Cancer in General," *Website Content*, 2001 www.bccancer.bc.ca/pg_t_03.asp?PageID=8&ParentID=2

Columbia University College of P & S Complete Home Medical Guide, "General Definition of Cancer," CPMCnet, Columbia Presbyterian Medical Center, *Website Content*, 2001 www.cpmcnet.columbia.edu/texts/guide/hmg17_0001.html

Fierro, M., "How Much Does Cancer Cost?", Nat. Governors Ass'n, NGA Center for Best Practice, *Website Content*, 2001 www.nga.org/center/divisions/1,1188,T_CEN_HES%5EC_ISS UE_BRIEF%5ED_1915,00.html

Foti, M., "Defeating Cancer – A Sense of Urgency and a Need for Strategic Continuity," American Association for Cancer Research, *Website Content*, March 2000 www.aacr.org/5000/5300/5300e.html

Gutman, H.A., "Review of Anti-Angiogenesis Drugs for Lung Cancer," *excerpt*, A Complete Guide to Lung Cancer, 2001 http://www.lungcancerclaims.com/antiangiogenis%20lung%20 cancer.htm

Health Canada, "Economic Burden of Illness in Canada, 1993," *Website Content*, 1997 www.hc-sc.gc.ca/hpb/lcdc/publicat/burden/order-e.html

Jacobs, T., "Five Promising Cancer Drugs," The Motley Fool, *Website Content*, 2001 www.fool.com/news/foth/2001/foth010618.htm

King, M.W., "DNA Synthesis," *The Medical Biochemistry Page*, Indiana State University, 2001 web.indstate.edu/thcme/mwking/dna.html

Memorial Sloan-Kettering Cancer Center, "Nausea and Vomiting," *Website Content*, 2001 www.mskcc.org/patients_n_public/about_cancer_and_treatment/ side_effects/nausea_and_vomiting_print.html

Minton, S.E., "New Hormonal Therapies for Breast Cancer," *Cancer Control*, Journal of the Moffitt Cancer Center, 6(3), May/June 1999   www.moffitt.usf.edu/pubs/ccj/v6n3/article3.htm

National Cancer Institute of Canada, "Canadian Cancer Statistics 2001," *Website Content*, 2001 www.cancer.ca/stats/highle.htm

Oncolink, University of Pennsylvania Cancer Center, National Cancer Institute Information Resources, "NCI Fact Sheet: Paclitaxel (Taxol) and Related Anticancer Drugs – Updated 02/2000," *Website Content*, 2001 cancer.med.upenn.edu/pdq_html/6/engl/600715.html

Ralph, S.J., Devenish, R.J., "Interferons as Cell Modulators in Health and Disease," Monash University, Australia, *Website Content*, 2000 www.med.monash.edu.au/biochem/research/projects/interferons.html

Roche Pharmaceuticals, "Roche Acquires Anti-Nausea and Vomiting Drug from SmithKline Beecham," Hoffman-La Roche Inc., *Website Content*, January 3, 2001 www.rocheusa.com/newsroom/current

Salvatore, S., The Associated Press, "FDA Panel Approves Potentially Powerful Breast Cancer Drugs," *Cable News Network*, September 1998 www.cnn.com/HEALTH/9809/02/breast.cancer.drug.03/

The Association of the British Pharmaceutical Industry, "Prostate Disease and the Pharmaceutical Industry," *Website Content*, 2001 www.abpi.org.uk/publications/publication_details/targetProstate/section5d.htm

The CancerBACUP Factsheet, "Flutamide (Drogenil)" *Website Content*, 1999 www.cancerbacup.org.uk/info/flutamide.htm

University of Nebraska Medical Center, Department of Pharmacology, "Cancer Basics, Characteristics of Cancer Cells," *Lecture Notes*, 2001 www.artemis.unmc.edu:82/cancer/canpath.htm

Aids/ HIV

AIDS Research Information Center, Inc., On-Line AIDS Medical Glossary: Retroviral Reproduction, *Website Content*, 2001 www.critpath.org/aric/gloss/body/retroviral_reproduction.htm

AIDS Treatment News, "ddI, d4T, Hydroxyurea: New Pancreatitis Warning," AIDS.ORG Inc., Issue 331, *Website Content*, 1999 www.immunet.org/immunet/atn.nsf/page/a-331-01

Blakeslee, D.J., "Entry Inhibitors: The More the Better," JAMA HIV/AIDS Resource Center, September 22, 2000 www.ama-assn.org/special/hiv/newsline/conferen/icaac00/dbentry.htm

Downs, M.F., "Adding to Antiretroviral Arsenal: New AIDS Drugs in Development," *CBS HealthWatch*, February 2001 cbshealthwatch.medscape.com/cx/viewarticle/234098_3

HealthCommunities.com, Inc., "Antiretroviral Therapy," *Website Content*, 2001 www.hivchannel.com/arvt/nonnuc.shtml

"HIV and AIDS in Canada, Surveillance Report to December 31, 2000," Centre for Disease Control, Health Protection Branch Health Canada, April 2001; "National Trends of AIDS and HIV in Canada," *Canada Communicable Disease Report*, 26(23), December 1, 2000 www.avert.org/canstatg.htm

JAMA, HIV/AIDS Resource Center, "Treatment Guidelines, HIV/AIDS Drugs Information," *Website Content*, 2000 www.ama-assn.org/special/hiv/treatmnt/druginfo/druginfo.htm

James, J.S., "Lipodystrophy: Glaxo Researchers Suggest Mechanisms," *AIDS Treatments News*, No. 315, 1999 www.immunet.org/Immunet/atn.nsf/page/a-315-01

Johns Hopkins AIDS Service, "Life Cycle of HIV Infection," Johns Hopkins University, *Website Content*, 2001 www.hopkins-aids.edu/hiv_lifecycle/hivcycle_txt.html

Markowitz, M., "Protease Inhibitors: What They Are, How They Work, When to Use Them," International Association of Physicians in AIDS Care, *Website Content*, 2000 www.iapac.org/clinmgt/avtherapies/patient/proinbk.html

Park, A., "The Hunt for Cures. AIDS, Still No Vaccine, but Better Antiviral Drugs Are on the Way," *Time Europe*, 157(2), January 15, 2000 www.time.com/time/europe/magazine/2001/0115/cover_cures.html

Pharmaceutical Research and Manufacturers of America, "AIDS and the Pharmaceutical Industry," *Website Content*, November 1998 www.phrma.org/publications/backgrounders/development/aids98.phtml

Shikuma, C., "What is Lactic Acidosis Syndrome and Mitochondrial Toxicity?" National AIDS Treatment Advocacy Project (NATAP), *Website Content*, 2000 www.natap.org/2000/lipo/lipo_rp4pt1whatislact092200.htm

The Canadian HIV/AIDS Clearinghouse, Canadian Public Health Association, *Website Content* www.clearinghouse.cpha.ca/english/about/hdoffice.htm

U.S. Department of Health and Human Services, Public Health Service, Centers for Disease Control and Prevention, National Center for HIV, STD and TB Prevention, "United States HIV & AIDS Statistics Summary," *HIV/AIDS Surveillance Report, Mid Year Edition*, 12(12), 2000 www.avert.org/statsum.htm

U.S. Department of Health and Human Services, National Center for Health Statistics, "AIDS/HIV," *Website Content*, 2001 www.cdc.gov/nchs/fastats/aids-hiv.htm

U.S. Department of Health and Human Services, National Institute of Allergy and Infectious Diseases, National Institutes of Health, Office of Communications and Public Liaison, Public Health Service, *Fact Sheet, HIV/AIDS Statistics*, 2001 www.niaid.nih.gov/factsheets/aidsstat.htm

U.S. FDA, "Approved Drugs for HIV/AIDS," *Website Content*, 2001 www.fda.gov/oashi/aids/stat_app.html

Additional Resources

Martindale's Health Science Guide – 2001
www-sci.lib.uci.edu/~martindale/Pharmacy.html

The Merck Manual of Diagnosis and Therapy
www.merck.com/pubs/mmanual/

Oncolink, University of Pennsylvania Cancer Center
cancer.med.upenn.edu/

Pharmaceutical News and Information
www.coreynahman.com/

Rxlist, the Internet Drug Index
www.rxlist.com/

Journal References

Manor, D., Sadeh, M., "Muscle Fiber Necrosis Induced by Intramuscular Injection of Drugs," *British Journal Experimental Pathology*, (4):457-462, 1989

Soni, S.D., Wiles, D., Schiff, A.A., Bamrah, J.S., "Plasma Levels of Fluphenazine Decanoate, Effects of Site Injection, Massage and Muscle Activity," *British Journal of Psychiatry*, 153:382 384, 1988

Ueda, W., Katatoka, Y., Sagara, Y., "Effect of Gentle Massage on Regression of Sensory Analgesia During Epidural Block," *Anaesthesia and Analgesia*, 76:783-5, 1993

Cardiovascular

Hennekens, C.H., Dyken, M.L., Fuster, V., "Aspirin as a Therapeutic Agent in Cardiovascular Disease," *Circulation*, 96:2751-2753, 1997, American Heart Association, Inc.

Saari, J.T., Dahlem, G.M., "Nitric Oxide and Cyclic GMP are Elevated in the Hearts of Copper-Deficient Rats," *Medical Science Research*, 26:495-497, 1998

Shafeer, R.S., Lacivita, C.L., "Choosing Drug Therapy for Patients with Hyperlipidemia," *American Academy of Family Physicians*, 61:3371-82, 2000

Diabetes

Linde, B., "Dissociation of Insulin Absorption and Blood Flow During Massage of a Subcutaneous Injection Site," *Diabetes Care*, 4(2):570-574, Nov-Dec, 1986

Emotional and Mood Disorders

Fried, I.,Wilson, C., Morrow, J.W., Cameron, K.A., Behnke, E.D., Ackerson, L.C., Maidment, N.T., "Increased Dopamine Release in the Human Amygdala During Performance of Cognitive Tasks," *Nature Neuroscience*, 4(2):201-206, February, 2001

Pazzagli, L., Banfi, R., Borselli, G., Semmola, M.V., "Photosensitivity Reaction to Fluoxetine and Alprazolam," *Pharmacy World Science*, 20(3):136, 1998

Cancer

Batchelor, T.T., Taylor, L.P., Posner, J.B., DeAngelis, L.M., "Steroid Myopathy in Cancer Patients," *Neurology*, 48(5):1234-8, May, 1997

Grover, S.A., Zowall, H., Coupal, L., Krahn, M.D., "Prostate Cancer: The Economic Burden," *CMA Journal*, 160:685-90, 1999 www.cma.ca/cmaj/vol-160/issue-5/0685.htm

Pain and Inflammation

Dvivedi S., Tiwari, S.M., Sharma, A., "Effect of Ibuprofen and Diclofenac Sodium on Experimental Wound Healing," *Indian Journal of Experimental Biology*, 35(11):1234-5 November, 1997

Eisenberg, D.M., Kessler, R.C., Foster, C., Norlock, F.E., Calkins, D.R., Delbanco, T.L., "Unconventional Medicine in the United States, Prevalence, Cost and Patterns of Use," *New England Journal of Medicine*, January 28, 1993

Flick, D.S., Johnson J.S, "Resolving Inflammation in Active Patients," *Physician and Sportmedicine*, 21(12), December, 1993

Johnson, A.G., "NSAIDs and Blood Pressure, Clinical Importance for Older Patients," *Drugs And Aging*, 12(1):17-27, January, 1998

Johnson, A.G., "NSAIDs and Increased Blood Pressure, What Is the Clinical Significance?" *Drug Safety*, 17(5):277-89, November, 1997

Lee, K.H., "Studies on the Mechanism of Action of Salicylate II. Retardation of Wound Healing by Aspirin," *Journal of Pharmacy Science*, 57(6):1042-43, June, 1968

McCormack, K., "The Spinal Actions of Nonsteroidal Drugs and the Dissociation Between their Anti-Inflammatory and Analgesis Effects," *Drugs*, 47:28-45, 1994

McGoldrick, M.D., Bailie, G.R., "Nonnarcotics Analgesics: Prevalence and Estimated Economic Impact of Toxicities," *Annals of Pharmacotherapy*, 31(2):221-7, February, 1997

Mishra, D.K., Friden, J., Schmitz, M.C., Lieber, R.L., "Anti-Inflammatory Medication After Muscle Injury. A Treatment Resulting in Short Term Improvement but Subsequent Loss of Muscle Function," *Journal of Bone and Joint Surgery-American*, 77:10, 1510-9, October, 1995

Nielsen, A.C., *Market Track*, supplied by the Nonprescription Drug Manufacturers Association of Canada

Petersen, K.l., Brennum, J., Dahl, J.B., "Experimental Evaluation of the Analgesic Effect of Ibuprofen on Primary and Secondary Hyperanalgesia," *Pain*, 70(2-3):167-74, April, 1997

Rapoport, A., Stang, P., Gutterman, D.L., Cady, R., Markley, H., Weeks, R., Saiers, J., Fox, A.W., "Analgesic Rebound Headache in Clinical Practice: Data from a Physician Survey," *Headache*, 36(1):14-9, January, 1996

Reynolds, J.K., Noakes, T.D., Schwellnus, M.P., et al., "Non-Steroidal Anti-Inflammatory Drugs Fail to Enhance Healing of Acute Hamstring Injuries Treated with Physiotherapy," *South African Medical Journal*, 85(6):517-22, June, 1995

Ruoff, G.E., "The Impact of Nonsteroidal Drugs on Hypertension: Alternative Analgesics for Patients at Risk," *Clinical Therapeutics*, 20(3):376-87, May-June, 1998

Sellman, J.R., "Plantar Fascia Rupture Associated with Corticosteroid Injection," *Foot & Ankle International*, 15(7):376-81, July, 1994

Wen, S.F., "Nephrotoxicities of Nonsteroidal Anti-Inflammatory Drugs," *Journal of the Formosan Medical Association*, 96(3):157-71, March, 1997

Wong, S.H., White, S., "Standards of Laboratory Practice: Analgesic Drug Monitoring. National Academy of Clinical Biochemistry," *Clinical Chemistry*, 44(5):1110-23, May, 1998

Ziegler, R., Kasperk, C., "Glucocorticoid-Induced Osteoporosis: Prevention and Treatment," *Steroids*, 63(5-6):344-8, May-June, 1998

Text References

Bates, B., *A Guide to Physical Examination and History Taking*, 5th ed., J.B. Lippincott, Philadelphia, 1991

Brodal, P., *The Central Nervous System*, Oxford University Press, New York. 1992

Boyle, W., Saine, A., *Lectures In Naturopathic Hydrotherapy*, Buckeye Naturopathic Press, Ohio, 1988

Canadian Pharmaceutical Association, *Compendium of Pharmaceutical Specialties*, 28th ed., Ottawa, 1993

Ciccone, C.D., *Pharmacology In Rehabilitation*, 2nd ed., F. A. Davis Company, Philadelphia, 1996

Curties, D., *Massage Therapy and Cancer*, Curties-Overzet Publications, Moncton, 1999

Donovan, E.D., *Essentials of Pathophysiology*, Macmillan Publishing Company, New York, 1985

Freeman Clarke, J.B., Queener, S.F., & Burke Karb, V., *Pharmacologic Basis of Nursing Practice*, 4th ed., Mosby Year Book Inc., Missouri, 1993

Gershon, M.D., *The Second Brain*, Harper Collins Publishers, New York, 1998

Goodman, C.C., Boissonnault, W.G., *Pathology: Implications for the Physical Therapist*, W.B. Saunders Company, Philadelphia, 1998

Kellogg, J.H., *Rational Hydrotherapy*, 4th ed., Modern Medicine Publishing Company, 1928

Kisner, C., Colby, L.A., *Therapeutic Exercises: Foundations and Techniques*, 3rd ed., F.A. Davis Company, Philadelphia, 1996

Lappe, M., *The Body's Edge*, Henry Holt & Company Inc., New York, 1996

Juhan, D., *Job's Body*, Station Hill Press Inc., New York, 1987

MacDermott, B.L., Deglin, J.H., *Understanding Basic Pharmacology: Practical Approaches for Effective Application*, F.A. Davis Company, Philadelphia, 1994

Magee, D.J., *Orthopedic Physical Assessment*, 3rd ed., W.B.Saunders Company, Philadelphia, 1997

Michlovitz, S.L., *Thermal Agents in Rehabilitation*, 3rd ed., F.A. Davis Company, Philadelphia, 1996

Moore, K.L., *Clinically Oriented Anatomy*, 2nd ed., Williams & Wilkins, Baltimore, 1985

Nolte, J., *The Human Brain*, 3rd ed., Mosby Year Book Inc., Missouri, 1993

Ramamurthy, S., Rogers, J.N., *Decision Making in Pain Management*, Mosby Year Book Inc., Missouri, 1993

Reynolds J.E.F, Prasad, A.B., eds., Martindale, *The Extra Pharmacopoeia*, 28th ed., The Pharmaceutical Press, London, 1982

Skidmore-Roth, L., *Mosby's Nursing Drug Reference*, Mosby Year Book Inc., Missouri, 1994

Smith C.M., Reynard, A.M., *Essentials of Pharmacology*, W.B. Saunders Company, Philadelphia, 1995

Tabers Cyclopedic Medical Dictionary, 16th ed. F.A. Davis Company, Philadelphia, 1989

United States Pharmacopeial Convention Inc., *USP DI, Drug Information for the Health Care Professional, Volume 1A*, 12th ed., Maryland, 1992.

United States Pharmacopeial Convention Inc., *USP DI, Drug Information for the Health Care Professional, Volume 1B*, 12th ed., Maryland, 1992

United States Pharmacopeial Convention Inc., *USP DI, Advice for the Patient, Volume 11*, 12th ed., Maryland, 1992

Vannini, V., Pogliani, G., *The Color Atlas Of Human Anatomy*, Beekman House, New York, 1980

Weintraub, W., *Tendon and Ligament Healing*, North Atlantic Books, California, 1999

Index

NOTE: Brand name medications are not indexed; use generic names.

3TC, 213

acarbose, 133
ACE inhibitors, 106–8, 118–19, 123
acetaminophen, 79, 80, 82
actinomycin D, 193
acyclovir, 213
adverse effects. See side effects
affective disorders, 163–84
age, 19, 26
agranulocytosis, 183
AIDS/HIV, 209–25
albumin, 39–40, 42, 142
albuterol, 151
alcohol, 138
alemtuzumab, 188
alitretinoin, 188
alkylating drugs, 193, 198, 200–1, 205
allergic reactions, 21, 148–50
allopathic medicine, 13
allopurinol sodium, 189
alpha-glucosidase inhibitors,
    133, 134, 135, 143
alpha receptor drugs, 107–8, 118–19
alprazolam, 167
amifostine, 188
aminolevulinic acid HCL, 189
amitriptyline, 170
amprenavir, 215
anaesthetics, 59, 71, 167
analgesics; see also narcotic analgesics
    57, 60, 63, 154
anaphylaxis reactions, 21
anastrozole, 188, 195
anemia, 159, 220
angina pectoris, 28–9, 97, 98, 124
angiogenesis inhibitors, 197–8
antacids, 17
antiandrogenic drugs, 195–6
anti-anxiety drugs,
    46, 55, 56, 58, 60, 85, 164, 165–8
antibiotics, 62, 64, 70
anticholinergic drugs, 150, 152
anticoagulants, 12, 56, 109–10, 118–19
anticonvulsants, 43–4
antidepressants, 46, 55, 164, 168–73
anti-emetic drugs, 199–200
antiestrogenic drugs, 195
antihistamines,
    148–9, 154, 155, 158–9, 161
antihypertensives,
    17, 46, 55, 58–9, 65, 79, 222

anti-inflammatories, 52, 57, 70
antimetabolites, 193, 198, 200–1, 205
antinausea drugs, 199–200
antineoplastic drugs, 192–8
antipsychotics, 164, 173–5
antithrombotics, 110–11
antitumor antibiotics,
    193–4, 198, 200–1, 206
antitussives, 154–5, 160
antiviral drugs, 213–17
anxiety, 163, 165–8
arsenic trioxide, 188
aspirin, 12–13, 24, 28, 38, 79, 82
    effects, 19, 20, 56, 146, 158
    uses, 18, 19, 50, 80, 111
assessment, 45–53, 66–8
asthma,
    63–5, 145–6, 150, 154, 157, 158, 161
atherosclerosis, 97, 98
Attention Deficit Hyperactivity Disorder
(ADHD), 59
atypical antipsychotics,
    175, 176–8, 182–3
AZT, 213

barbiturates, 167
BCG, live, 188
benzodiazepines,
    164, 167, 168, 176–8, 182, 183, 184
benzonatate, 154
beta-adrenergic agonists, 151, 152
beta blockers,
    17, 18, 101–3, 118–19, 122
bexarotene, 189
bicalutamide, 195
biguanides, 132–3, 134, 135, 142
bile acid sequestrants, 116
bioavailability, 26
biological response modifiers, 187
bipolar depression, 169
bleomycin, 189, 193
blood brain barrier (BBB), 40–1
blood coagulation, 56, 109–12, 123
blood disorders, 220
blood flow, 39
blood pressure, 99–100
body tissues, 51, 56–7, 157
brain, 39, 40–1
brand names, 15–16
bronchitis, 145–6, 154, 161
bronchodilators, 150–2, 155, 159
bruising, 56
buserelin, 195
buspirone HC1, 167–8, 176–8
busulfan, 188, 193

cabergoline, 189
caffeine, 17, 152
calcium channel blockers,
    17, 51–2, 65, 105–6, 108, 118–19, 123
cancer, 185–208
capecitabine, 188
captopril, 107
carbamazepine, 43–4
cardiac dysrhythmia, 97, 98
cardiac glycosides, 103–4, 118–19
cardiovascular disease, 97–124
cardizen, 106
carmustine wafer, 188
case history taking, 47–51
    cancer, 202
    cardiovascular disease, 120
    diabetes, 139
    HIV/AIDS, 218
    injection sites, 66–7
    mood disorders, 179
    pain and inflammation, 91
    respiratory conditions, 156
catheters, implanted; see also implant
    devices, 34–5, 36
celecoxib, 188
cell cycle, 190–2
centrally acting skeletal muscle
    relaxants, 12, 52, 56, 85
central venous catheter (CVC), 34–5
cerebrovascular accident, 98
chemical drug names, 15
chemical structure, 17–18
chemotherapy, 187–9
chilled client, 61
chloral hydrate, 167
chlorambucil, 193
chloropromazine, 174
chloropropramide, 132
chlorpheniramine, 148
chlorpromazine, 200
cholesterol, 115–17
chronic obstructive pulmonary disease
(COPD), 145–6
chronic pain, 54
client complaints, 45–6
client cooperativeness, 58
client feedback, 55
clonidine, 108, 189
clozapine, 175
CNS depressants,
    17, 52, 55, 60, 63, 85, 95
CNS stimulants, 17, 59
codeine, 60, 81, 82, 160
combining of therapies, 13, 43
common flu, 50, 62

congestion, 59, 145–61, 153–4
congestive heart failure, 98, 103, 124
constitution, 19
contraceptives, 33, 73
corticosteroids, 12, 18, 50, 52, 60, 62, 86–9, 94, 95, 138, 153–4, 160, 195
  side effects, 46, 55, 56, 89–90
cortisone type injections, 65
cough and cold medications, 154
cough suppressants, 154–5, 160
coumarin derivatives, 109
counter-irritants, 30, 93
Crohn's disease, 41
cromolyn sodium, 150, 155, 159
cyclobenzaprine, 12, 85
cyclophosphamide, 193
cytarabine, 189, 193

d4T, 213
dacarbazine, 193
Dantrolene, 85, 90
daunorubicin, 188, 193
ddC, 213
ddI, 213
decongestants, 59, 153, 154, 155, 159, 160, 161
deep vein thrombosis, 206
delavirdine, 214
denileukin diftitox, 189
depots, 33
depression, 163, 164, 168–73
dermal administration; see skin applications
dexamethasone, 12, 199, 200
dextroamphetamine, 59
dextromethorpham hydrobromide (DM), 154, 160
diabetes, 54, 64, 125–44
diabetic coma, 136–7
diabetic instability, 136–8
diarrhea, 41, 207
diazepam, 19, 20, 167
diclofenac, 79
didanosine, 213
digitalis, 103–4, 122
digitoxin, 103
digoxin, 103
dimenhydrinate, 200
diphenhydramine, 148, 154, 199
dipyridamole, 111
dissolving and dissociating, 37–8
diuretics, 17, 65, 113–14, 118–19, 123
docetaxel, 188
dolasetron mesylate, 189, 199
dopamine, 164, 168, 172, 173, 175
dosage, 19, 26, 38
doxazosin, 108
doxorubicin, 189, 193
droperidol, 200
drug classification, 16–18

drug distribution, 39–41
drug names, 15–16
drug processing, 37–42
drug pumps, 34, 35–6, 129–30
dysthymia, 169

ear drops, 29
efavirenz, 214
effects; see also side effects 17, 19–21
elimination, 41–2
Elliotts B Solution, 189
embolus, 98
emotional disorders, 163–84
emotional stability, 55
emphysema, 145–6, 161
enalapril, 107
enteric coated preparations, 28
entry inhibitors, 216
ephedrine, 59
epidural block, 65
epilepsy, 44, 54, 167
epinephrine HC1, 151
epirubicin hydrochloride, 188
ergot alkaloid derivatives, 108
estrogen, 194–5
etoposide phosphate, 188
excipients, 37, 41
exemestane, 188
exercise, 63–5, 138
  with cancer, 207–8
  with cardiovascular disease, 124
  with diabetes, 143–4
  with HIV/AIDS, 224
  with mood disorders, 184
  with pain and inflammation, 95
  with respiratory conditions, 161
expectorants, 153, 154, 155, 160
experimental uses, 18
eye drops, 29

fasting, 42, 138
fatigue, 55
fenoterol hydrobromide, 151
fentanyl citrate, 189
fever, 70, 71, 157
fibric acid derivatives, 116–17
filgrastim, 188
first pass effect, 38, 39
floxuridine, 193
fludarabine, 193
fludeoxyglucose, 189
fluorouracil, 193
fluoxetine, 172
fluphenazine decanoate, 65
flutamide, 195
frequency of administration, 26

gamma-aminobutyric acid (GABA), 164, 167, 168
garlic, 142

gastrointestinal disorders, 38, 41
gemcitabine HCL, 188, 189
gemtuzumab ozogamicim, 188
generic drugs, 15, 16, 41
glipizide, 132
glycosuria, 125
goserelin, 189, 195
granisetron, 189, 199, 200
griseofulvin, 38
guaifenesin, 153

half-life, 25
haloperidol, 174, 200
heart attack, 63, 97, 98, 124
heart rate, 100–1
heavy tapotement, 157
heparin, 109, 110
histamine, 148
HIV/AIDS, 209–25
HMG Co A reductase inhibitors, 116–17
hormonal agents, 194–6, 198, 200–1, 206
hydrocodone, 81
hydrotherapy, 12, 58–62, 71–2
  with cancer, 206–7
  with cardiovascular disease, 124
  with diabetes, 143
  with HIV/AIDS, 223–4
  with mood disorders, 175, 183
  with pain and inflammation, 95
  with respiratory conditions, 160–1
hydroxyzine, 200
hyperemia, 12
hyperglycemia, 123, 125, 136–8, 223
hyperlipidemia, 115–16
hypersensitivity reactions, 21
hypertension, 50, 58–9, 62, 63, 64, 97, 98, 100, 222
hypoglycemia, 136–8, 141, 142
hypotension, 59, 122, 160
hypothermia, 175

ibuprofen, 12–13, 52, 79, 158
idarubicin, 193
imatinib mesylate, 188
immunocompromised clients; see also HIV/AIDS, 70, 140
immunotherapy, 187
implant devices, 65–70, 72
implanted catheters, 34–5, 36
"indications," 18–19
indinavir, 215
infants, 71
inflammation, 79–90
injections, 32–3, 129
injection sites, 32–3, 52, 65–72, 141–2
insomnia, 138
insulin, 54, 65, 72, 125, 127–31, 135, 138
insulin shock, 136–7

interactions among medications, 19, 21, 50, 51, 79, 138, 142
interferons, 189, 196–7, 198, 200–1, 206, 215, 216
intestinal paralysis, 206
intra-arterial injections, 32
intra-articular injections, 32, 33, 69
intradermal injections, 32
intralesional injections, 32
intramuscular injections, 32, 33, 39, 69, 71
intrathecal injections, 32
intravenous administration, 26, 32, 39, 69, 71
ipratropium bromide, 152
irinotecan hydrochloride, 188

joint pain, 30

Kaposi's sarcoma, 188, 215
ketazolam, 38, 167
kidney dysfunction, 25, 122
kidneys, 39, 41–2, 44, 50, 204
kidney stones, 222

lactic acidosis, 214, 221–2
lamivudine, 213
letrozole, 188
letter to medical practioner, 53
leukemia, 188
leukopenia, 220
leuprolide acetate, 189
LHRH analogs, 195–6
lipid lowering drugs, 115–19, 123
lipid soluble drugs, 41, 65
lipodystrophy, 215, 223
lipoproteins, 115–16
liquid oral preparations, 27, 28, 37
lisinopril, 107
lithium, 172–3, 176–8, 183, 184
liver, 38, 39, 41–2, 44, 50, 204
liver dysfunction, 25, 220
long-term drug use, 50–1, 52, 62, 95
loop diuretics, 114
lopinavir/ritonavir, 215
lorazepam, 167
lungs, 39, 41, 145
luteinizing hormone, 195
lymphoma, 189

manic-depressive disorder, 169
manual technique selection, 56–8
massage therapy
  defined, 12
  vs. pharmacy, 12
mechanisms of action, 22–5
mechlorethamine, 193
meclizine, 200
medical stability, 54, 64–5, 140
metabolism, 38–9
metformin, 132

methotrexate, 193
methoxsalen, 189
methyldopa, 108
methylphenidate, 59
metoclopramide, 200
metoprolol, 102
migraine, 59
mitotic spindle drugs, 194, 198, 200–1, 206
mitoxantrone hydrochloride, 189
mood disorders, 163–84
morphine, 81
mother's milk, 41
movement examination, 52, 68
mucous membrane applications, 28–9
multiple sclerosis, 63
muscle pain, 30
muscle spasm, 84
mustard poultices, 161
myocardial infarction; see heart attack

nadolol, 102
naproxen, 79
narcotic analgesics, 17, 18, 52, 81–3, 94, 95, 160
  side effects, 55, 56, 58, 59, 90
nausea, 199
nefazodone, 172
nelfinavir, 215
nerve block, 32
neuritis, 159
neurological tests, 52
neurotransmitters, 163–4
neutropenia, 220
nevirapine, 214
niacin, 116–17
nicotine patch, 73
nicotinic acid, 116–17
nifedipine, 106
nilutamide, 189, 195
nitroglycerine, 28–9, 31, 39, 73, 104, 123
non-nucleoside reverse transcriptase inhibitors (NNRTIs), 214, 216, 217, 222
non-steroidal anti-inflammatory drugs; see NSAIDs
norepinephrine, 164, 170–1, 172, 173
NSAIDs, 12–13, 18, 24, 28, 79–81, 94, 95, 111, 142
  side effects, 46, 55, 56, 90, 146, 158
nucleoside analogues reverse transcriptase inhibitors (NRTIs), 213–14, 216, 217, 221–2, 223, 224

observation, 51–2, 67
obsessive-compulsive disorder, 166
octreotide acetate, 189
odansetron, 189, 199
olanzapine, 175
ondansetron, 200
onset of action, 25–6

ophthalmic administration, 29
opiates; see narcotic analgesics
oprelvekin, 189
oral administration, 27–8
oral hypoglycemic drugs, 131–4, 142–3
osteoporosis, clients at risk for, 57, 94
otic administration, 29
over-the-counter medications, 47, 79, 154
oxtriphylline, 151
oxymetazoline, 153

paclitaxel, 188, 189, 194
pain, 79–90
pain perception, 52, 57
palpation, 52, 67
pamiddronate disodium, 188
pancreas, 125
pancreatitis, 220
panic disorder, 166
paralytic ileus, 206
parenteral administration; see also injections, 31–3
paresthesias, 124, 142, 159, 182
Parkinson's Disease, 164
paroxetine, 172
pathologies, 19, 26, 38
perineural injections, 32
peripheral neuropathy, 205, 214, 221, 223
perphenazine, 200
pethidine, 81
petrissage, 12
pharmacology, defined, 11
pharmacy, vs. massage therapy, 12
phenothiazines, 12, 60, 64, 174–5, 176–8, 182, 183, 184
phobias, 166
photosensitivity reactions, 64
pioglitazone, 133
plasma protein binding, 39–40, 42
platelet inhibitors, 56
plicamycin, 193
post-traumatic stress disorder, 166
potassium iodide, 153
potassium sparing diuretics, 114
prazosin, 108
prochlorperazine, 199, 200
profimer sodium, 188
propranolol, 102
protease inhibitors (PIs), 215, 216, 217, 222–3, 224
protective responses, 56
pseudoephedrine, 59, 153
psychosis, 173–5
pulmonary fibrosis, 205, 206

radiation therapy, 186–7, 207
referrals, 46, 53
renin-angiotensin system, 106–7

resource texts, 13–14
respiratory inflammation, 145–61
retroviruses, 210
reverse transcriptase inhibitors, 213–14, 216
risperidone, 175
ritonavir, 215
rituximab, 189
rosiglitazone, 133
routes of administration, 26, 27–36

samarium, 189
saquinavir, 215
schizophrenia, 173–4
scopolamine, 200
seasonal affective disorder, 169
selective serotonin re-uptake inhibitors (SSRIs), 172–3, 176–8, 182, 183, 184
self care, 63
serotonin, 164, 168, 170–1, 172, 173, 175
sertindole, 175
sertraline, 172
side effects, 19–20, 21, 46
  of cancer drugs, 200–1
  of cardiovascular drugs, 118–19
  of diabetes drugs, 135
  of HIV/AIDS drugs, 214, 215, 217
  at injection sites, 69
  of mood disorder drugs, 176–8
  of pain and inflammation drugs, 90
  of respiratory drugs, 155
sinus infection, 62
skeletal muscle relaxants, 12, 52, 56, 63, 64, 84–6, 90, 94, 95
skin, 39, 57, 60, 220
skin applications, 30–1, 60, 65–70, 93
skin patches, 31, 73
sleep disorders, 138, 164
solid oral preparations, 27–8, 37, 41
solubility, 41
spasticity, 84
special tests, 52
starch blockers; see alpha-glucosidase inhibitors
statins, 116–17
stavudine, 213
streptokinase, 112
stroke, 63, 97, 124
subcutaneous injections, 32, 33
sublingual administration, 39
succinyl-choline, 85, 86
sulfa drugs, 64
sulfonylureas, 132, 134, 135, 142, 143
sumatriptan, 59
suppositories, 39

tamoxifen, 188, 195, 206
temozolomide, 189
testosterone, 194–5
theophylline, 151

thiazide diuretics, 114, 138
thiazolidinediones (TZDs), 133–6, 143
thiethylperazine, 200
thrombocytopenia, 220
thrombolytics, 112
thrombophlebitis, 71
thrombus, 98, 111
timed release preparations, 28
timolol, 102
tissue plasminogen activator (tPA), 112
topical applications, 29–31
topotecan hydrochloride, 188, 189
toremifene, 188, 195
toxicity, 44, 122, 173, 183, 204
transient ischemic attack, 98
trastuzumab, 188
treatment guidelines; see also case history taking; exercise; hydrotherapy 43–58, 74–5
  for cancer, 203–8
  for cardiovascular disease, 121–4
  for diabetes, 140–4
  for HIV/AIDS, 219–25
  for injection sites, skin applications, and implant devices, 65–73
  for mood disorders, 180–4
  for pain and inflammation, 92–5
  for respiratory conditions, 157–61
treatment planning, 54–8
treatment scheduling, 54–5
tricyclic antidepressants, 170–2, 176–8, 182, 183, 184
trifluoperazine, 12, 174
triglycerides, 115–17
triptorelin pamoate, 189
troglitazone, 133
tubulin inhibitors, 194
typical antipsychotics, 174–5

ulcers, 38, 41

vaccinations, 71
valrubicin, 188
vasoconstriction, 58–60
vasodilation, 12, 58–60, 104–8, 222
vasodilators, 12, 17, 65, 104–5, 108, 118–19, 123
venlafaxine, 172
verapamil, 106
vinblastine, 194
vincristine, 194
viral replication, 210–12
vitamin K, 109–10
vomiting, 41, 199, 207

warfarin, 109, 110

xanthine derivatives, 151, 152

zalcitabine, 213
zidovudine, 213
zoledronic acid, 189

great website for older adults.
NIHseniorhealth.gov.